HEART DISEASE COOKBOOK FOR WOMEN

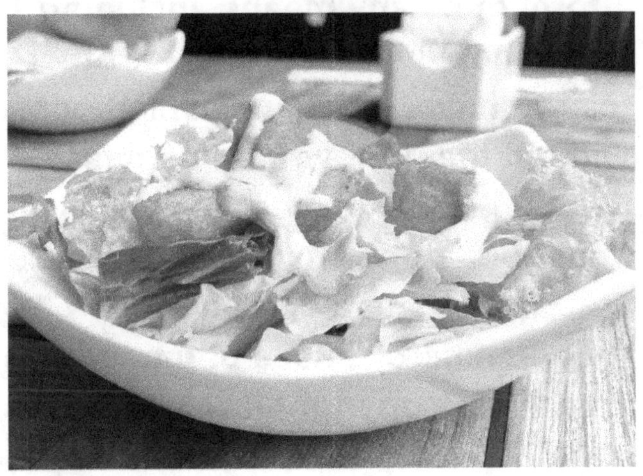

"Nourishing Her Heart: A Culinary Journey to Women's Cardiovascular Wellness, With Over 30 Delicious And Healthy Recipe"

EMMA LYNCH

TABLE OF CONTENTS

INTRODUCTION

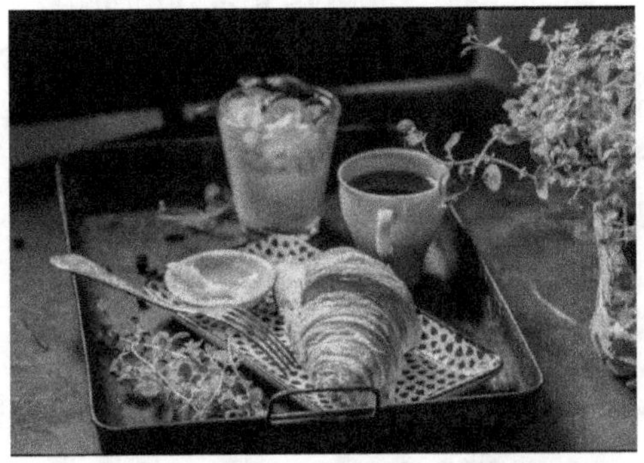

Welcome to the "Heart Disease Cookbook For Women" In the pages that follow, we embark on a culinary exploration specifically designed to address the unique aspects of heart health in women. Heart disease is a formidable adversary, and this cookbook serves as a compassionate guide, empowering women to take control of their well-being through the art of mindful and heart-conscious cooking.

In a world where the demands on women are diverse and dynamic, prioritizing cardiovascular health is paramount. This cookbook is more than a collection of recipes; it's a holistic approach to nurturing your heart. We recognize that women's heart health requires a nuanced understanding, and each recipe within these pages is crafted with care to support your journey toward a healthier, heartful life.

From breakfasts that set a heart-healthy tone for the day to satisfying dinners that prioritize nutrient-rich ingredients, we aim to make every meal a step toward wellness. Alongside delicious recipes, we provide insights into the role of essential nutrients, mindful cooking techniques, and lifestyle practices that contribute to a heart-conscious existence.

So, let the Heart Disease Cookbook For Women be your companion in creating meals that not only delight your taste buds but also fortify your heart. Here's to nourishing your heart, embracing well-being, and savoring the journey towards a healthier you.

CHAPTER ONE

UNDERSTANDING HEART HEALTH

Understanding heart health is essential for fostering overall well-being and preventing cardiovascular diseases, which remain a leading cause of mortality globally. The heart, a powerful muscle, plays a central role in the circulatory system, pumping blood rich in oxygen and nutrients to all parts of the body.

1. Anatomy and Function:
   Two atria and two ventricles make up the four chambers of the heart. Atria receive blood, while ventricles pump it out. The cardiac cycle involves rhythmic contractions and relaxations, ensuring a continuous flow of blood. Understanding this dynamic process is fundamental to appreciating the heart's vital role in sustaining life.

2. Risk Factors:
   Recognizing risk factors is crucial for heart health. High blood pressure, elevated cholesterol levels, smoking, diabetes, and a sedentary lifestyle are common contributors to heart disease. Genetic factors also play a role, underlining the importance of personalized health assessments.

3. Lifestyle Choices:

Adopting heart-healthy habits significantly influences cardiovascular well-being. Regular physical activity strengthens the heart, improves circulation, and helps manage weight. A balanced diet, rich in fruits, vegetables, whole grains, and lean proteins, contributes to optimal heart function.

4. Nutritional Impact:

Nutrition is a cornerstone of heart health. Understanding the impact of nutrients is vital. Omega-3 fatty acids, found in fish and nuts, contribute to heart health by reducing inflammation and supporting blood vessel function. Fiber helps lower cholesterol, while antioxidants from fruits and vegetables protect against oxidative stress.

5. Monitoring and Prevention:

Regular health check-ups, including blood pressure and cholesterol screenings, enable early detection and intervention. Prevention involves maintaining a healthy weight, managing stress, limiting alcohol intake, and avoiding tobacco.

6. Age and Gender Considerations:

Age and gender influence heart health. Women may experience unique heart disease symptoms, and risk factors may vary at different life stages. Understanding these nuances ensures tailored preventive measures.

7. Holistic Approach:

Heart health is not solely about physical factors; emotional well-being matters too. Stress management, quality sleep, and a supportive social network contribute to a holistic approach to heart health.

In conclusion, understanding heart health is a multifaceted endeavor encompassing anatomy, risk factors, lifestyle choices, nutrition, monitoring, and a holistic perspective. Armed with this knowledge, individuals can make informed decisions, take proactive measures, and cultivate habits that promote a resilient and thriving heart throughout life.

IMPORTANCE OF NUTRITION IN PREVENTING HEART DISEASE

Nutrition plays a pivotal role in preventing heart disease, serving as a powerful tool for maintaining cardiovascular health. The choices we make in our diets directly impact risk factors associated with heart-related conditions. Here's a breakdown of the importance of nutrition in preventing heart disease:

1. Cholesterol Management:
   Dietary choices influence cholesterol levels, a key factor in heart health. Saturated and trans fats, commonly found in processed foods and certain animal products, can raise LDL (low-density lipoprotein) cholesterol. On the other hand,

incorporating heart-healthy fats, such as those found in olive oil, avocados, and nuts, can help manage cholesterol levels.

2. Blood Pressure Regulation:
One of the biggest risk factors for heart disease is high blood pressure. A diet rich in potassium (found in fruits, vegetables, and legumes) and low in sodium can help regulate blood pressure. The DASH (Dietary Approaches to Stop Hypertension) diet, for example, emphasizes these principles for blood pressure control.

3. Weight Management:
A healthy weight is essential for heart health. Nutrient-dense, whole foods contribute to satiety, making it easier to manage weight. Additionally, a diet high in fiber, found in fruits, vegetables, and whole grains, supports weight management by promoting feelings of fullness.

4. Diabetes Prevention and Management:
Diabetes increases the risk of heart disease. Choosing complex carbohydrates, monitoring sugar intake, and maintaining a balanced diet can help prevent and manage diabetes, subsequently reducing the risk of cardiovascular complications.

5. Antioxidant Protection:
Antioxidants, abundant in fruits and vegetables, protect the heart by neutralizing free radicals that contribute to inflammation and damage to blood

vessels. Berries, leafy greens, and colorful
vegetables are rich sources of these protective
compounds.

6. Omega-3 Fatty Acids for Heart Health:
   Omega-3 fatty acids, found in fatty fish,
flaxseeds, and walnuts, have anti-inflammatory
properties and support heart health. Including these
sources in the diet helps reduce the risk of heart
disease by promoting optimal lipid profiles and
maintaining blood vessel health.

7. Overall Heart-Healthy Patterns:
   Diets that emphasize a variety of nutrient-dense
foods, limit processed and sugary items, and
include a balance of macronutrients contribute to
overall heart health. Mediterranean and
plant-based diets, for instance, have been
associated with a lower risk of heart disease.

In essence, nutrition serves as a cornerstone in
preventing heart disease. Making informed and
heart-conscious food choices can positively impact
cholesterol levels, blood pressure, weight, and
overall cardiovascular well-being. A balanced and
nutrient-rich diet, complemented by a healthy
lifestyle, is a potent strategy for cultivating a heart
that thrives in the face of preventive measures.

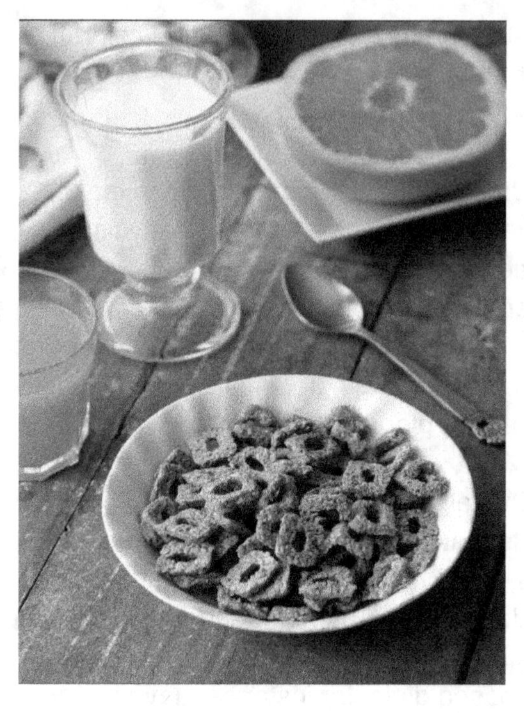

CHAPTER TWO

HEART-HEALTHY BASICS

Heart-Healthy Basics: Nurturing Cardiovascular Wellness

In the realm of heart health, adopting fundamental principles sets the stage for a resilient cardiovascular system. The "Heart-Healthy Basics" section of this cookbook provides a foundation for crafting meals that prioritize well-being. Let's explore these essential elements:

ESSENTIAL NUTRIENTS FOR CARDIOVASCULAR HEALTH

Essential Nutrients for Cardiovascular Health: A Comprehensive Guide

Maintaining cardiovascular health relies heavily on incorporating key nutrients into your diet. These essential elements play distinct roles in supporting heart function, regulating cholesterol levels, and promoting overall well-being.

1. Omega-3 Fatty Acids:
  - **Sources:** Fatty fish (salmon, mackerel, trout), flaxseeds, chia seeds, walnuts.

- **Benefits:** Omega-3s are renowned for their anti-inflammatory properties. They contribute to a healthy heart by reducing blood clotting, improving blood vessel function, and lowering triglyceride levels. Regular consumption is associated with a decreased risk of heart disease.

2. Fiber:
- **Sources:** Whole grains (oats, barley, quinoa), fruits (apples, berries, pears), vegetables (broccoli, Brussels sprouts), legumes.
- **Benefits:** Fiber is a multifaceted nutrient crucial for heart health. It helps lower LDL (bad) cholesterol levels, regulates blood sugar, and promotes a feeling of fullness, aiding in weight management. It also helps to maintain a healthy digestive tract.

3. Potassium:
- **Sources:** Bananas, oranges, potatoes, sweet potatoes, leafy greens (spinach, kale).
- **Benefits:** Potassium is essential for maintaining proper blood pressure levels. It counteracts the effects of sodium, helping to regulate fluid balance and reduce strain on the heart. Adequate potassium intake is associated with a lower risk of stroke and cardiovascular events.

4. Antioxidants:

- **Sources:** Berries (blueberries, strawberries), citrus fruits, dark chocolate, nuts (especially almonds), spinach.
- **Benefits:** Antioxidants neutralize free radicals in the body, reducing oxidative stress and inflammation. This protection is vital for preventing damage to blood vessels and decreasing the risk of atherosclerosis.

Understanding the significance of these nutrients involves not only incorporating them into your diet but also ensuring a diverse and balanced intake. Consider adopting a variety of foods rich in omega-3 fatty acids, fiber, potassium, and antioxidants to create a nutrient-packed foundation for cardiovascular wellness. A diet that encompasses these essential nutrients contributes not only to heart health but also to overall vitality and longevity.

COOKING TECHNIQUES FOR HEART-FRIENDLY MEALS

Cooking Techniques for Heart-Friendly Meals: A Detailed Exploration

Creating heart-healthy meals extends beyond ingredient choices; it involves thoughtful consideration of cooking methods. The right techniques can enhance flavors, preserve nutritional integrity, and contribute to overall cardiovascular wellness.

1. Grilling:
   - **Principles:** Grilling allows for the preparation of flavorful meals without excessive added fats.
   - **Heart-Friendly Tips:** Choose lean proteins like skinless poultry, fish, or plant-based alternatives. Marinate with heart-healthy herbs and spices to add flavor without relying on excessive salt or saturated fats.

2. Roasting:
   - **Principles:** Roasting uses high heat to cook food, preserving nutrients and enhancing natural flavors.
   - **Heart-Friendly Tips:** Roast a variety of colorful vegetables and lean proteins like chicken or turkey. Incorporate heart-healthy oils, such as olive oil, for added richness.

3. Steaming:
   - **Principles:** Steaming retains the maximum nutritional value of foods by cooking them with steam.
   - **Heart-Friendly Tips:** Steam a variety of vegetables, fish, or poultry for a light and nutrient-packed meal. Add heart-healthy herbs and citrus for extra flavor.

4. Sautéing:

  - **Principles:** Sautéing involves cooking food quickly in a small amount of heart-healthy oil.
  - **Heart-Friendly Tips:** Use oils rich in monounsaturated fats, such as olive oil, for sautéing. Combine colorful vegetables, lean proteins, and whole grains for a balanced and heart-conscious dish.

5. Baking:
  - **Principles:** Baking is a gentle cooking method that allows for the retention of nutrients.
  - **Heart-Friendly Tips:** Bake whole grains, fish, or skinless poultry with herbs and spices for added flavor. Opt for whole-grain flours in baking for increased fiber content.

6. Poaching:
  - **Principles:** Poaching involves gently simmering food in liquid, preserving moisture.
  - **Heart-Friendly Tips:** Poach fish, poultry, or eggs with flavorful broths or water infused with herbs. This method imparts subtle flavors without relying on added fats.

By embracing these heart-friendly cooking techniques, you not only enhance the taste and texture of your meals but also contribute to a heart-conscious lifestyle. Experiment with these methods, incorporating a variety of nutrient-dense foods, to create a diverse and satisfying menu that prioritizes cardiovascular wellness without compromising on culinary enjoyment.

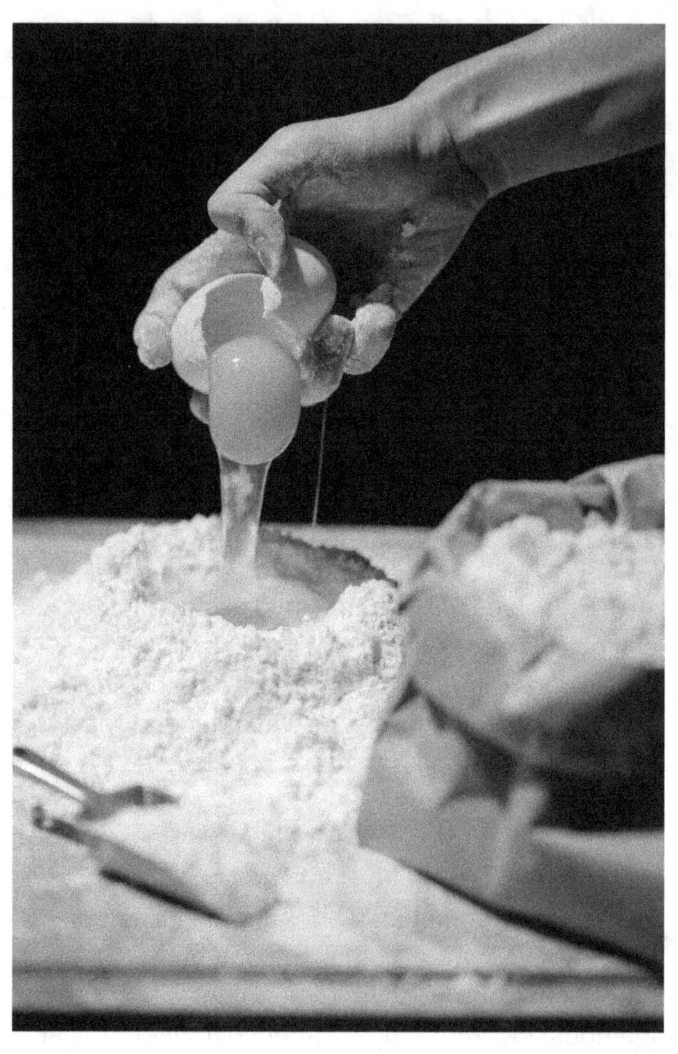

CHAPTER THREE

BREAKFAST BOOSTERS

"Breakfast boosters" refers to a collection of nutritious and energizing foods that are specifically chosen to provide a positive start to your day. These breakfast options are designed to boost your energy, provide essential nutrients, and support overall well-being. The term encompasses a variety of wholesome ingredients and meal ideas that go beyond mere sustenance, aiming to kickstart your metabolism, enhance focus, and set a healthy tone for the rest of the day.

Typically, breakfast boosters include a balance of macronutrients (carbohydrates, proteins, and fats), as well as essential vitamins and minerals. Examples may include:

1. **Protein-rich options:** Eggs, Greek yogurt, lean meats, or plant-based proteins like nuts and seeds. Protein helps with satiety and muscle repair.

2. **Fiber-packed foods:** Whole grains, fruits, and vegetables contribute fiber, promoting digestive health and providing a sustained release of energy.

3. **Healthy fats:** Avocado, nuts, seeds, and olive oil can add heart-healthy fats, supporting brain function and helping you feel satisfied.

4. **Antioxidant-rich fruits:** Berries, citrus fruits, and other colorful options provide antioxidants, which combat oxidative stress and support overall health.

5. **Hydrating beverages:** Water, herbal teas, or fresh fruit juices can contribute to hydration, essential for optimal bodily functions.

Whether it's a smoothie with nutrient-dense ingredients, a balanced oatmeal bowl, or a protein-packed egg dish, breakfast boosters aim to maximize nutritional value to fuel your body and mind. Incorporating a variety of these elements into your morning routine can help you feel more alert, satisfied, and ready to tackle the day ahead.

FIBER-RICH MORNING STARTERS

Certainly! Here are 5 fiber-rich morning starter recipes with detailed instructions:

1. **Quinoa Breakfast Bowl:

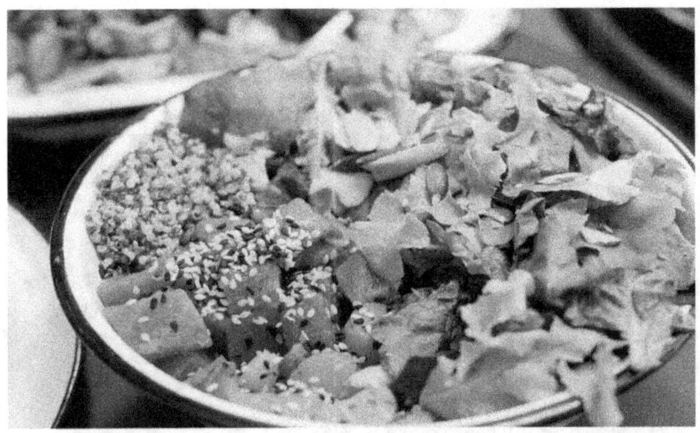

Certainly! Here's a nutritious and tasty recipe for a Quinoa Breakfast Bowl:

Ingredients:

- 1 cup cooked quinoa
- Half a cup of almond milk, or any other type of milk.
- 1 tablespoon honey or maple syrup
- 1/2 teaspoon vanilla extract
- Fresh fruits (such as berries, sliced banana, or mango)
- Nuts and seeds (such as almonds, chia seeds, or pumpkin seeds)
- Greek yogurt or coconut yogurt
- Optional toppings: cinnamon, nutmeg, or shredded coconut

Instructions:

Prepare Quinoa:
  - Cook quinoa according to package instructions.
You can use water or a mix of water and almond
milk for added flavor.

 Sweeten Quinoa:
  - In a bowl, combine the cooked quinoa with
almond milk, honey (or maple syrup), and vanilla
extract. Stir well to combine.

Assemble Breakfast Bowl:
  - Spoon the sweetened quinoa into a breakfast
bowl.

Add Fresh Fruits:
  - Top the quinoa with an assortment of fresh
fruits, such as berries, sliced banana, or mango.

Add Nuts and Seeds:
  - Sprinkle your choice of nuts and seeds over the
fruits for added crunch and nutrition. Almonds, chia
seeds, and pumpkin seeds work well.

Include Yogurt:
  - Add a dollop of Greek yogurt or coconut yogurt
to the bowl. This adds creaminess and protein.

Optional Toppings:
  - Sprinkle cinnamon, nutmeg, or shredded
coconut on top for additional flavor.

Enjoy:

- Mix everything together or leave it layered for a visually appealing breakfast. Enjoy your wholesome and customizable Quinoa Breakfast Bowl!

Feel free to get creative with your toppings, adjusting them based on your taste preferences and what's in season. This breakfast bowl is not only delicious but also packed with protein, fiber, and a variety of nutrients to kickstart your day.

2. Overnight Chia Seed Pudding:

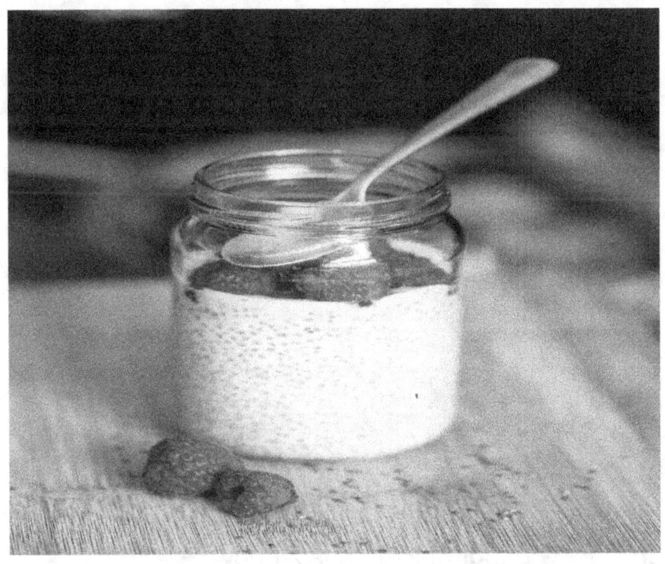

Certainly! Here's a simple and delicious recipe for Overnight Chia Seed Pudding:

Ingredients:

- 1/4 cup chia seeds
- One cup almond milk, or any other type of milk you prefer
- One tablespoon honey or maple syrup, adjusted to taste
- 1/2 teaspoon vanilla extract
- Fresh fruits (berries, sliced banana, or mango) for topping
- Nuts and seeds (almonds, sliced almonds, or pumpkin seeds) for topping
- Optional: a sprinkle of cinnamon or a dash of nutmeg

Instructions:

Mix Ingredients:
  - In a bowl or jar, combine chia seeds, almond milk, maple syrup (or honey), and vanilla extract. Make sure the chia seeds are dispersed evenly by giving it a good stir.

Refrigerate Overnight:
  - Cover the bowl or jar and refrigerate the mixture overnight or for at least 4-6 hours. This enables the liquid to be absorbed by the chia seeds, giving the mixture a pudding-like consistency.

Stir Before Serving:

- The next morning or when ready to eat, give the pudding a good stir to break up any clumps and achieve a smooth texture.

Top with Fresh Fruits and Nuts:
   - Spoon the chia seed pudding into a serving bowl or glass.
   - Top with fresh fruits and nuts of your choice. Berries, sliced banana, and almonds are classic choices.

Optional Toppings:
   - Sprinkle a bit of cinnamon or a dash of nutmeg on top for extra flavor.

Enjoy:
   - Grab a spoon and enjoy your nutritious and delicious Overnight Chia Seed Pudding!

This recipe is not only versatile but also a great option for a quick and convenient breakfast or snack. The chia seeds provide omega-3 fatty acids, fiber, and protein, making it a satisfying and healthy choice. You are welcome to alter the toppings to suit your tastes.

3. High-Fiber Smoothie:

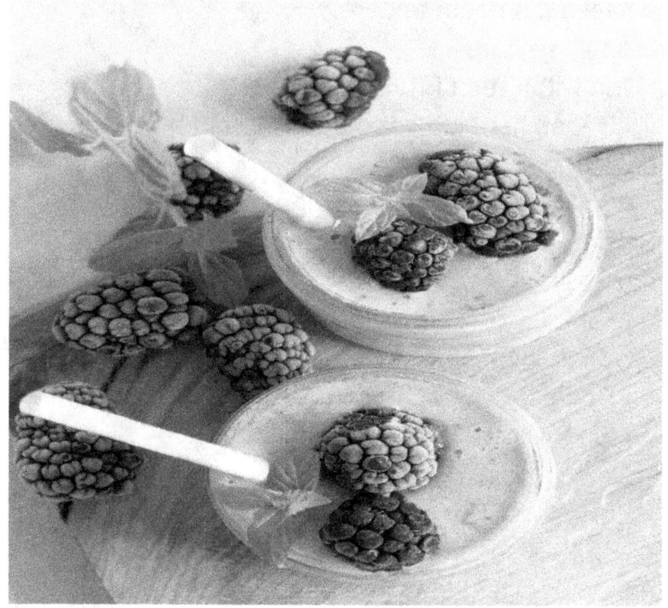

Absolutely! Here's a recipe for a High-Fiber Smoothie that's both delicious and packed with nutritional goodness:

Ingredients:

- 1 cup spinach (fresh or frozen)
- 1/2 cup kale (fresh or frozen)
- 1/2 cup frozen berries (blueberries, strawberries, or a mix)
- 1/2 banana (fresh or frozen)
- 1 tablespoon chia seeds
- 1 tablespoon ground flaxseed

- Half a cup of plant-based or Greek yogurt
- 1 cup almond milk or any milk of your choice
- One tsp honey or maple syrup (to taste, optional)
- Ice cubes (optional)

Instructions:

Combine Ingredients:
   - In a blender, combine spinach, kale, frozen berries, banana, chia seeds, ground flaxseed, Greek yogurt, and almond milk.

Sweeten (Optional):
   - If you want more sweetness, you can add honey or maple syrup. Keep in mind that the sweetness from the fruits and yogurt might be sufficient.

Blend:
   - Mix every item until it becomes creamy and smooth. To get the right consistency, you can add more almond milk if the smoothie is too thick.

Adjust Thickness:
   - If you prefer a thicker consistency, you can add ice cubes and blend again until smooth.

Pour and Enjoy:
   - Pour the high-fiber smoothie into a glass and enjoy immediately.

This smoothie is not only rich in fiber but also provides a variety of vitamins, minerals, and antioxidants. Feel free to customize the ingredients based on your preferences and what you have available. It's a great way to start your day or as a healthy snack anytime!

4. Banana-Walnut Oatmeal:

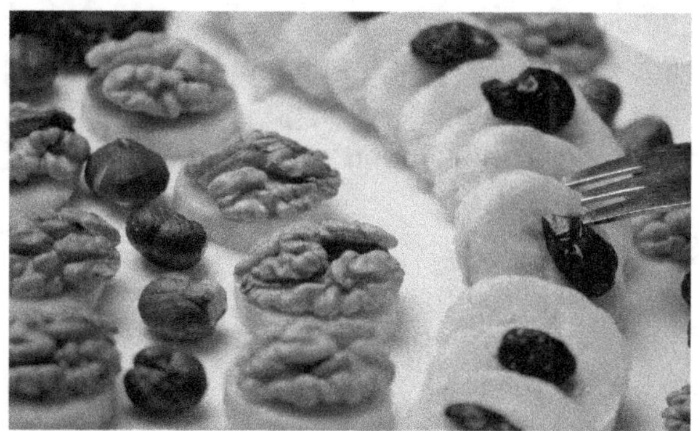

 Certainly! Here's a simple and hearty recipe for Banana-Walnut Oatmeal:

Ingredients:

- 1/2 cup old-fashioned rolled oats
- 1 cup milk (dairy or plant-based)
- 1 ripe banana, mashed
- 1/4 cup chopped walnuts
- One tablespoon of optionally sweetened maple syrup or honey
- 1/2 teaspoon vanilla extract
- Pinch of cinnamon (optional)
- Pinch of salt

- Sliced banana and additional walnuts for topping (optional)

Instructions:

Combine Oats and Milk:
   - In a saucepan, combine rolled oats and milk. Add a pinch of salt.

Cook Oatmeal:
   - Bring the mixture to a gentle boil over medium heat, then reduce the heat to a simmer.

Add Mashed Banana:
   - Stir in the mashed banana and continue to cook, stirring occasionally, until the oats are tender and the mixture has thickened to your liking.

Add Walnuts and Flavorings:
   - Stir in the chopped walnuts, honey or maple syrup (if using), vanilla extract, and a pinch of cinnamon if desired.

 Adjust Sweetness and Texture:
   - Taste the oatmeal and adjust sweetness or add more milk if needed to reach your desired consistency.

Serve:
   - Spoon the Banana-Walnut Oatmeal into a bowl.

Top and Enjoy:

  - Top with additional sliced banana and walnuts if desired.

Serve Warm:
  - Serve the oatmeal warm and enjoy a comforting and nutritious breakfast!

This Banana-Walnut Oatmeal is not only delicious but also provides a good balance of carbohydrates, fiber, and healthy fats. Feel free to add more fruits or your preferred toppings to make it uniquely yours. It's a wholesome and satisfying way to start your day!

5. Mixed Berry Parfait:

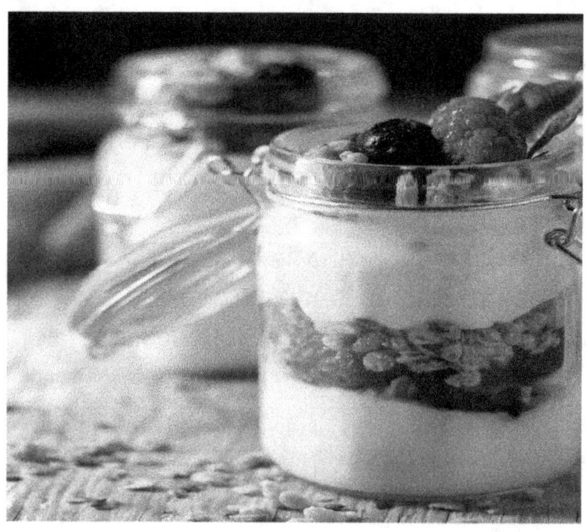

Certainly! Here's a delightful recipe for a Mixed Berry Parfait:

Ingredients:

- One cup of mixed berries, including raspberries, blueberries, and strawberries
- 1 cup Greek yogurt or vanilla yogurt
- 1/2 cup granola
- One tablespoon of maple syrup or honey (optional, to be drizzled on)
- Fresh mint leaves for garnish (optional)

Instructions:

Prepare Berries:
  - Wash and slice any larger berries like strawberries.

Layer Yogurt:
  - Start by adding a spoonful of Greek yogurt to the bottom of serving glasses or bowls.

Add Berries:
  - Spread some mixed berries over the yogurt.

Sprinkle Granola:
  - Top the berries with a coating of granola.

Repeat Layers:

- Repeat the layers until you reach the top of the glass or bowl, finishing with a layer of berries on top.

 Drizzle with Honey (Optional):
   - For extra sweetness, you can pour some honey or maple syrup on top if you'd like.

Garnish:
   - Garnish with fresh mint leaves for a burst of freshness.

Serve:
   - Serve the Mixed Berry Parfait immediately and enjoy!

This Mixed Berry Parfait is not only visually appealing but also a delicious and nutritious treat. It's rich in antioxidants, fiber, and protein. Feel free to customize the parfait with your favorite fruits or switch up the yogurt flavor. It's a versatile and refreshing option for breakfast or a healthy dessert!

These fiber-rich morning starters are not only delicious but also packed with nutrients to keep you fueled and satisfied throughout the day. Enjoy a variety of flavors while boosting your daily fiber intake for optimal digestive health.

LOW-SODIUM AND NUTRIENT-PACKED OPTIONS

Certainly! Here are 4 low-sodium and nutrient-packed recipes along with detailed instructions:

1. **Grilled Lemon Herb Salmon:

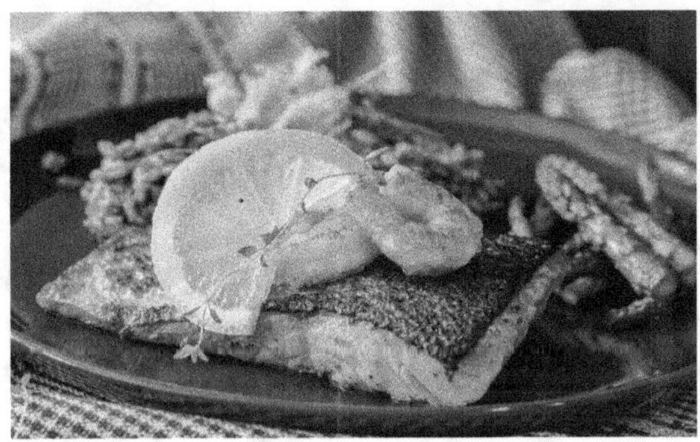

Certainly! Here's a simple and flavorful recipe for Grilled Lemon Herb Salmon:

Ingredients:

- Four 6-ounce salmon fillets
- 2 tablespoons olive oil
- 2 tablespoons fresh lemon juice
- 2 cloves garlic, minced
- 1 teaspoon fresh thyme, chopped
- 1 teaspoon fresh rosemary, chopped
- 1 teaspoon fresh parsley, chopped
- Salt and black pepper to taste

- Lemon slices for garnish

Instructions:

Preheat Grill:
  - Turn the heat up to medium-high on your grill.

Prepare Marinade:
  - In a small bowl, whisk together olive oil, fresh lemon juice, minced garlic, chopped thyme, rosemary, parsley, salt, and black pepper.

Marinate Salmon:
  - Place the salmon fillets in a shallow dish or a zip-top bag. Make sure every fillet of salmon has a good coating by pouring the marinade over them. Allow the flavors to infuse by marinating for a minimum of 15 to 30 minutes.

Oil Grill Grates:
  - Brush the grill grates with a bit of oil to prevent sticking.

Grill Salmon:
  - Place the marinated salmon fillets on the preheated grill, skin side down. Close the lid and grill for about 4-6 minutes per side, or until the salmon easily flakes with a fork. Depending on the thickness of the fillets, cooking times can change.

Check for Doneness:

- Salmon is done when it easily flakes but is still moist in the center. Be cautious not to overcook to keep it juicy.

Garnish and Serve:
   - Place the salmon that has been grilled on a serving plate. Garnish with lemon slices and additional fresh herbs if desired.

Serve Warm:
   - Serve the Grilled Lemon Herb Salmon warm and enjoy your flavorful and healthy meal!

This Grilled Lemon Herb Salmon is not only delicious but also a great source of omega-3 fatty acids and protein. It's a perfect dish for a light and satisfying dinner. Feel free to pair it with your favorite grilled vegetables or a side salad.

2. **Quinoa and Vegetable Stir-Fry:

Certainly! Here's a tasty and nutritious recipe for Quinoa and Vegetable Stir-Fry:

Ingredients:

- 1 cup quinoa, rinsed
- 2 cups water or vegetable broth
- 2 tablespoons soy sauce
- 1 tablespoon sesame oil
- 1 tablespoon olive oil
- 2 cloves garlic, minced

- 1 tablespoon ginger, grated
- 1 cup broccoli florets
- 1 medium carrot, julienned
- 1 bell pepper (any color), thinly sliced
- 1 cup snap peas, ends trimmed
- 1 cup mushrooms, sliced
- Salt and black pepper to taste
- Green onions, chopped, for garnish
- Sesame seeds for garnish (optional)

Instructions:

Cook Quinoa:
  - In a saucepan, combine quinoa and water or vegetable broth. After bringing to a boil, lower the heat to a simmer, cover, and let the quinoa cook for approximately 15 minutes, or until the liquid has been absorbed.

 Prepare Stir-Fry Sauce:
  - In a small bowl, mix soy sauce and sesame oil. Set aside.

Sauté Aromatics:
  - In a large skillet or wok, warm the olive oil over medium-high heat. Add minced garlic and grated ginger, sautéing for about 1 minute until fragrant.

Stir-Fry Vegetables:
  - Add broccoli, julienned carrot, sliced bell pepper, snap peas, and mushrooms to the skillet. Sauté the

veggies for five to seven minutes, or until they are crisp-tender.

Combine Quinoa and Sauce:
   - Add cooked quinoa to the skillet, pouring the prepared soy sauce and sesame oil mixture over the top. Toss everything together until well combined.

Season:
   - Season with salt and black pepper to taste. Adjust the seasoning as needed.

Garnish:
   - Garnish the quinoa and vegetable stir-fry with chopped green onions and sesame seeds if desired.

 Serve:
   - Serve the Quinoa and Vegetable Stir-Fry warm and enjoy your wholesome and flavorful dish!

This Quinoa and Vegetable Stir-Fry is a versatile and satisfying option for a quick and healthy meal. Feel free to customize the vegetables based on your preferences, and you can also add tofu, chicken, or shrimp for added protein.

3. **Mango Avocado Chickpea Salad:

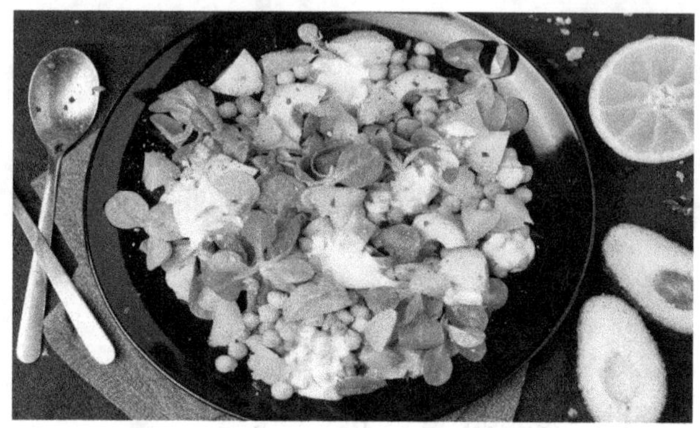

Certainly! Here's a refreshing and nutritious recipe for Mango Avocado Chickpea Salad:

Ingredients:

- 1 can (15 oz) chickpeas, drained and rinsed
- 1 ripe mango, diced
- 1 avocado, diced
- 1/2 red onion, finely chopped
- 1 red bell pepper, diced
- 1/4 cup fresh cilantro, chopped
- Juice of 1 lime
- 2 tablespoons olive oil
- Salt and black pepper to taste
- Optional: 1 jalapeño, seeded and finely chopped for a hint of spice

Instructions:

Prepare Chickpeas:
  - Drain and rinse chickpeas. If desired, you can pat them dry with a paper towel to remove excess moisture.

Combine Ingredients:
  - In a large bowl, combine chickpeas, diced mango, diced avocado, chopped red onion, diced red bell pepper, and chopped cilantro.

Make Dressing:
  - Mix the lime juice, olive oil, salt, and black pepper in a small bowl. If you like a bit of heat, you can add finely chopped jalapeño to the dressing.

Dress the Salad:
  - Pour the dressing over the chickpea and mango mixture. Mix everything together gently until evenly covered.

Chill (Optional):
  - You can refrigerate the salad for about 15-30 minutes to allow the flavors to meld, or serve it immediately.

Serve:
  - Serve the Mango Avocado Chickpea Salad on its own as a light meal or as a side dish to complement grilled proteins.

Enjoy:

- Enjoy this vibrant and flavorful salad that combines the sweetness of mango, creaminess of avocado, and the protein-packed chickpeas!

Feel free to adjust the quantities or add other ingredients like cherry tomatoes or cucumber to suit your taste preferences. This salad is not only delicious but also a great source of fiber, vitamins, and healthy fats.

4. **Roasted Vegetable Quinoa Bowl:

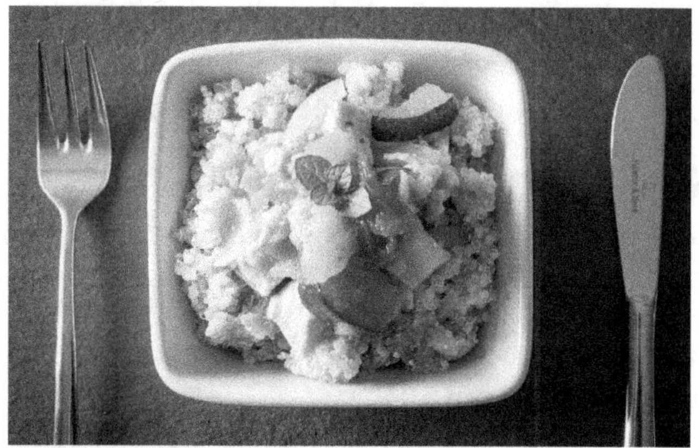

 Absolutely! Here's a delicious recipe for a Roasted Vegetable Quinoa Bowl:

Ingredients:

For Roasted Vegetables:
- 1 cup cherry tomatoes, halved
- 1 zucchini, sliced
- 1 bell pepper (any color), sliced
- 1 red onion, sliced

- 2 tablespoons olive oil
- 1 teaspoon dried thyme
- 1 teaspoon dried oregano
- Salt and black pepper to taste

For Quinoa:
- 1 cup quinoa, rinsed
- 2 cups vegetable broth or water
- 1 tablespoon olive oil
- 1 teaspoon lemon zest
- Salt to taste

For Lemon-Tahini Dressing:
- 2 tablespoons tahini
- 2 tablespoons lemon juice
- 1 tablespoon olive oil
- 1 clove garlic, minced
- Salt and black pepper to taste

Optional Toppings:
- Feta cheese crumbles
- Fresh parsley, chopped
- Avocado slices

Instructions:

Preheat Oven:
   - Set the oven temperature to 400°F, or 200°C.

Roast Vegetables:
   - In a large bowl, toss halved cherry tomatoes, sliced zucchini, bell pepper, and red onion with

olive oil, dried thyme, dried oregano, salt, and black pepper. Spread the vegetables on a baking sheet in a single layer and roast in the preheated oven for about 20-25 minutes or until they are tender and slightly caramelized.

 Cook Quinoa:
   - In a saucepan, combine quinoa and vegetable broth or water. After bringing to a boil, lower the heat to a simmer, cover, and let the quinoa cook for approximately 15 minutes, or until the liquid has been absorbed. Fluff with a fork and stir in olive oil, lemon zest, and salt.

 Prepare Lemon-Tahini Dressing:
   - In a small bowl, whisk together tahini, lemon juice, olive oil, minced garlic, salt, and black pepper. If necessary, thin the consistency with a small amount of water.

Assemble Bowls:
   - Divide the cooked quinoa among serving bowls. Top with the roasted vegetables.

 Drizzle with Dressing:
   - Pour in Lemon-Tahini. dressing to go with the roasted veggies and quinoa.

 Add Toppings:
   - Optional: Sprinkle feta cheese crumbles, chopped fresh parsley, and avocado slices on top.

Enjoy:
 - Enjoy your flavorful and nutritious Roasted
Vegetable Quinoa Bowl!

This bowl is not only colorful and visually appealing
but also provides a great balance of vegetables,
protein from quinoa, and a burst of flavor from the
lemon-tahini dressing. Feel free to customize the
recipe with your favorite vegetables and toppings.

These low-sodium and nutrient-packed recipes
offer delicious and wholesome options that
prioritize heart health and overall well-being.

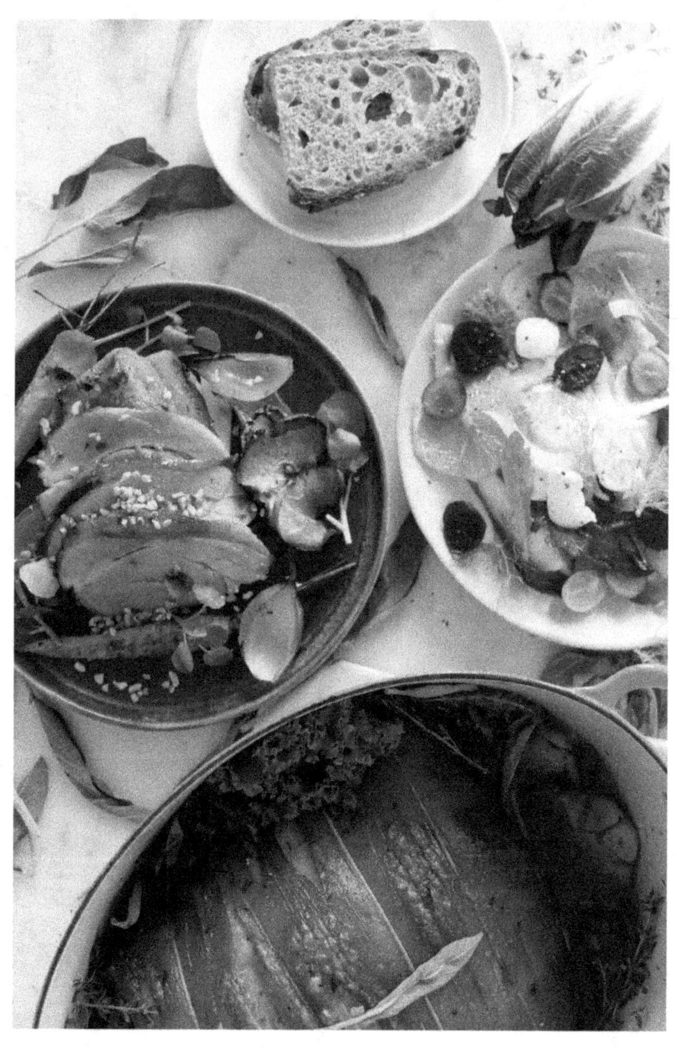

CHAPTER FOUR

LUNCHTIME DELIGHTS

"Lunchtime delights" refers to a variety of satisfying and enjoyable meals designed to make the midday dining experience a pleasurable and nourishing one. These dishes are not only flavorful but also thoughtfully crafted to provide a balanced mix of nutrients, energy, and taste.

Lunchtime delights can encompass a wide range of options, catering to various dietary preferences and culinary styles. They often focus on incorporating fresh and wholesome ingredients to create meals that not only satiate hunger but also contribute to overall well-being. The term emphasizes the idea that lunch can be a delightful and rewarding break during the day, offering an opportunity to enjoy delicious food that fuels the body and mind for the afternoon ahead.

Examples of lunchtime delights might include vibrant salads with a variety of colorful vegetables, whole-grain wraps filled with lean proteins and fresh produce, hearty soups packed with nutritious ingredients, or creatively assembled grain bowls that combine different textures and flavors.

Ultimately, lunchtime delights celebrate the idea that lunch can be more than just a necessity; it can be a moment to savor delicious and healthful food that brings joy and satisfaction to the daily routine. Whether prepared at home or enjoyed at a favorite lunch spot, these meals aim to make the midday break a delightful and nourishing experience.

LEAN PROTEINS AND HEART-HEALTHY FATS

Certainly! Here are 4 recipes featuring lean proteins and heart-healthy fats, along with detailed instructions:

1. Grilled Lemon Herb Chicken with Avocado Salsa:

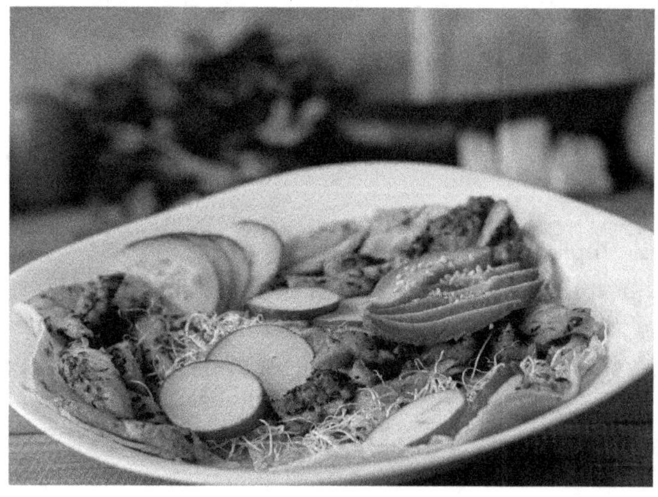

Certainly! Here's a delicious recipe for Grilled Lemon Herb Chicken with Avocado Salsa:

Ingredients:

For Grilled Lemon Herb Chicken:
- 4 boneless, skinless chicken breasts
- 2 tablespoons olive oil
- Zest of 1 lemon
- Juice of 1 lemon
- 2 cloves garlic, minced
- 1 teaspoon dried thyme
- 1 teaspoon dried rosemary
- Salt and black pepper to taste

For Avocado Salsa:
- 2 ripe avocados, diced
- 1 cup cherry tomatoes, halved
- 1/4 cup red onion, finely chopped
- 1/4 cup fresh cilantro, chopped
- Juice of 1 lime
- Salt and black pepper to taste

Instructions:

For Grilled Lemon Herb Chicken:

Preheat Grill:
   - Set the temperature of your grill to medium-high.

Prepare Chicken:

- In a bowl, combine olive oil, lemon zest, lemon juice, minced garlic, dried thyme, dried rosemary, salt, and black pepper.

Marinate Chicken:
- Put the chicken breasts in a zip-top bag or a shallow dish. Pour the marinade over the chicken, making sure each breast is well-coated. Marinate for at least 30 minutes.

Grill Chicken:
- Grill the chicken breasts for about 6-8 minutes per side or until they are cooked through and have nice grill marks. Depending on the thickness of the chicken, cooking times can change.

Rest and Slice:
- Before slicing, let the grilled chicken rest for a few minutes.

For Avocado Salsa:

Prepare Avocado Salsa:
- In a bowl, combine diced avocados, cherry tomatoes, red onion, cilantro, lime juice, salt, and black pepper. Gently toss to combine.

Serve:
- Serve the grilled lemon herb chicken slices topped with the flavorful avocado salsa.

Garnish (Optional):

- Garnish with additional cilantro or a squeeze of fresh lime juice if desired.

Enjoy:
   - Enjoy your Grilled Lemon Herb Chicken with Avocado Salsa for a burst of citrusy and herby flavors!

This recipe offers a perfect balance of grilled chicken with the freshness of avocado salsa. It's a light and vibrant dish that's easy to prepare and full of delicious, wholesome ingredients.

2. Baked Salmon with Dill Yogurt Sauce:

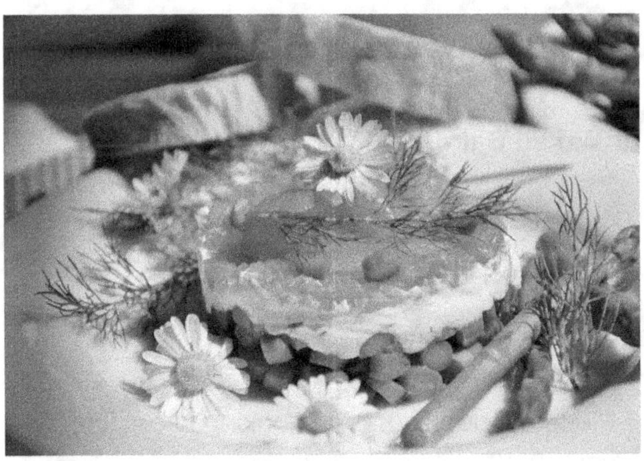

Certainly! Here's a delightful recipe for Baked Salmon with Dill Yogurt Sauce:

Ingredients:

For Baked Salmon:
- 4 salmon fillets
- 2 tablespoons olive oil
- 1 tablespoon lemon juice
- 2 cloves garlic, minced
- 1 teaspoon dried dill
- Salt and black pepper to taste
- Lemon slices for garnish (optional)

For Dill Yogurt Sauce:
- 1/2 cup Greek yogurt
- 1 tablespoon fresh dill, chopped
- 1 tablespoon lemon juice
- Salt and black pepper to taste

Instructions:

For Baked Salmon:

Preheat Oven:
   - Adjust the oven's temperature to 200°C, or 400°F.

Prepare Salmon:
   - Place salmon fillets on a baking sheet lined with parchment paper or lightly greased.

Make Marinade:
   - In a small bowl, whisk together olive oil, lemon juice, minced garlic, dried dill, salt, and black pepper.

Coat Salmon:
   - Brush the salmon fillets with the marinade,
making sure they are well-coated on both sides.

Bake Salmon:
   - Bake in the preheated oven for about 12-15
minutes or until the salmon easily flakes with a fork.
Depending on the thickness of the fillets, cooking
times can change.

Garnish (Optional):
   - Garnish with lemon slices if desired.

For Dill Yogurt Sauce:

Prepare Sauce:
   - In a small bowl, combine Greek yogurt, chopped
fresh dill, lemon juice, salt, and black pepper. Mix
until well combined.

Serve:
   - Serve the baked salmon fillets with a dollop of
dill yogurt sauce on top.

Garnish (Optional):
   - Garnish with additional fresh dill for extra flavor.

4. **Enjoy:**
   - Enjoy your Baked Salmon with Dill Yogurt
Sauce, a delicious and healthy meal!

This recipe provides a perfect balance of flavors with the herb-infused baked salmon and the creamy dill yogurt sauce. It's a simple yet elegant dish that's sure to impress!

3. Quinoa Salad with Chickpeas and Avocado:

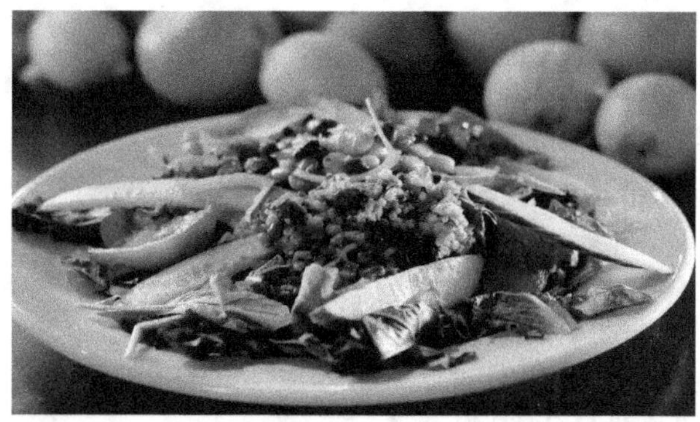

Certainly! Here's a tasty recipe for Quinoa Salad with Chickpeas and Avocado:

Ingredients:

- 1 cup quinoa, rinsed
- 2 cups water or vegetable broth
- 1 can (15 oz) chickpeas, drained and rinsed
- 1 ripe avocado, diced
- 1 cup cherry tomatoes, halved
- 1/4 cup red onion, finely chopped

- 1/4 cup fresh cilantro, chopped
- 1/4 cup feta cheese, crumbled (optional)
- 2 tablespoons olive oil
- 2 tablespoons lemon juice
- 1 clove garlic, minced
- Salt and black pepper to taste

Instructions:

Cook Quinoa:
- In a saucepan, combine quinoa and water or vegetable broth. After bringing to a boil, lower the heat to a simmer, cover, and let the quinoa cook for approximately 15 minutes, or until the liquid has been absorbed. Using a fork, fluff and allow to cool.

Prepare Chickpeas and Vegetables:
- In a large bowl, combine chickpeas, diced avocado, cherry tomatoes, red onion, and chopped cilantro.

Add Quinoa:
- Add the cooked and cooled quinoa to the bowl with chickpeas and vegetables.

Make Dressing:
- In a small bowl, whisk together olive oil, lemon juice, minced garlic, salt, and black pepper.

Combine and Toss:
- Transfer the dressing onto the combination of quinoa. Toss everything together until well coated.

Optional: Add Feta Cheese:
   - If using feta cheese, sprinkle it on top of the
salad and mix lightly.

Chill (Optional):
   - Refrigerate the quinoa salad for about 15-30
minutes to let the flavors meld, or serve it
immediately.

 Serve:
   - Serve the Quinoa Salad with Chickpeas and
Avocado as a refreshing and nutritious dish.

This quinoa salad is not only a great source of
protein and fiber but also bursting with fresh and
vibrant flavors. It's a versatile dish that works well
as a side or a light main course. You are welcome
to personalize it by adding your preferred herbs or
veggies.

4. Turkey and Spinach Stuffed Portobello Mushrooms:

 Certainly! Here's a delicious recipe for Turkey and
Spinach Stuffed Portobello Mushrooms:

Ingredients:

- 4 large Portobello mushrooms, stems removed
- 1 pound ground turkey
- 1 cup fresh spinach, chopped

- 1/2 cup onion, finely chopped
- 2 cloves garlic, minced
- 1/2 teaspoon dried thyme
- 1/2 teaspoon dried oregano
- Salt and black pepper to taste
- 1 cup cherry tomatoes, halved
- 1/2 cup feta cheese, crumbled
- Olive oil for drizzling
- Fresh parsley, chopped, for garnish (optional)

Instructions:

Preheat Oven:
   - Set oven temperature to 375°F, or 190°C.

Prepare Portobello Mushrooms:
   - Clean the Portobello mushrooms and remove the stems. Place them on a baking sheet, gill side up.

Sauté Turkey and Vegetables:
   - In a skillet, cook ground turkey over medium heat until browned. Add chopped onion, minced garlic, and chopped spinach. Cook until the onion is softened, and the spinach is wilted.

Season:
   - Season the turkey mixture with dried thyme, dried oregano, salt, and black pepper. Stir to combine.

Assemble Mushrooms:

- Spoon the turkey and vegetable mixture into each Portobello mushroom cap, pressing down gently.

 Add Toppings:
   - Top each stuffed mushroom with halved cherry tomatoes and crumbled feta cheese.

Drizzle with Olive Oil:
   - Drizzle olive oil over the stuffed mushrooms for added moisture.

Bake:
   - Bake in the preheated oven for about 20-25 minutes or until the mushrooms are tender and the toppings are golden brown.

Garnish (Optional):
   - Garnish with fresh chopped parsley if desired.

Serve:
   - Serve the Turkey and Spinach Stuffed Portobello Mushrooms warm and enjoy your flavorful and nutritious meal!

This recipe offers a satisfying and low-carb option with the earthy flavor of Portobello mushrooms complemented by the seasoned turkey and vibrant vegetables. Feel free to customize the stuffing ingredients based on your preferences.

These recipes provide a balance of lean proteins and heart-healthy fats, making them delicious and nutritious options for your meals.

CREATIVE SALADS AND SATISFYING SOUPS

Certainly! Here are 3 recipes for creative salads and satisfying soups, each with detailed instructions:

1. Quinoa and Chickpea Salad:

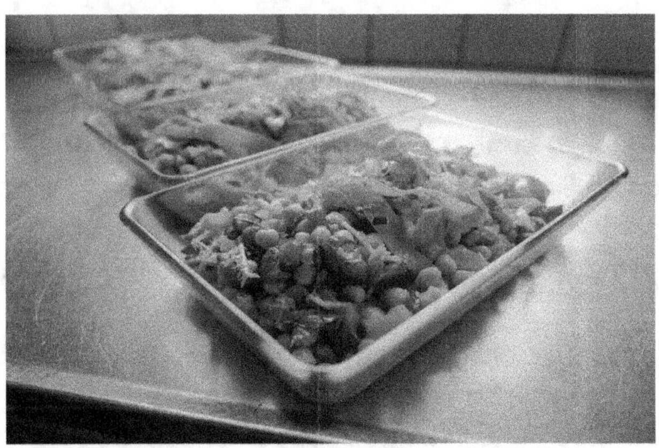

 Certainly! Here's a simple and nutritious recipe for Quinoa and Chickpea Salad:

Ingredients:

- 1 cup quinoa, rinsed

- 2 cups water or vegetable broth
- 1 can (15 oz) chickpeas, drained and rinsed
- 1 cucumber, diced
- 1 red bell pepper, diced
- 1/4 cup red onion, finely chopped
- 1/4 cup fresh parsley, chopped
- 1/4 cup feta cheese, crumbled (optional)
- 2 tablespoons olive oil
- 2 tablespoons lemon juice
- 1 teaspoon Dijon mustard
- 1 clove garlic, minced
- Salt and black pepper to taste

Instructions:

Cook Quinoa:
   - In a saucepan, combine quinoa and water or vegetable broth. After bringing to a boil, lower the heat to a simmer, cover, and let the quinoa cook for approximately 15 minutes, or until the liquid has been absorbed. Using a fork, fluff and allow to cool.

Prepare Chickpeas and Vegetables:
   - In a large bowl, combine chickpeas, diced cucumber, diced red bell pepper, chopped red onion, and chopped fresh parsley.

Add Quinoa:
   - Add the cooked and cooled quinoa to the bowl with chickpeas and vegetables.

Make Dressing:

- In a small bowl, whisk together olive oil, lemon juice, Dijon mustard, minced garlic, salt, and black pepper.

Drizzle and Toss:
  - Drizzle the dressing over the quinoa and chickpea mixture. Toss everything together until well coated.

Add Feta Cheese (Optional):
  - Crumble in the feta cheese, if using, and toss the salad lightly.

 Chill (Optional):
  - Refrigerate the quinoa and chickpea salad for about 15-30 minutes to let the flavors meld, or serve it immediately.

Serve:
  - Serve the Quinoa and Chickpea Salad as a refreshing and protein-packed dish.

This salad is not only delicious but also a great source of plant-based protein, fiber, and various nutrients. It's versatile and can be served as a side dish, light lunch, or a healthy main course. Feel free to customize it with your favorite vegetables or herbs.

2. Roasted Vegetable and Lentil Salad:

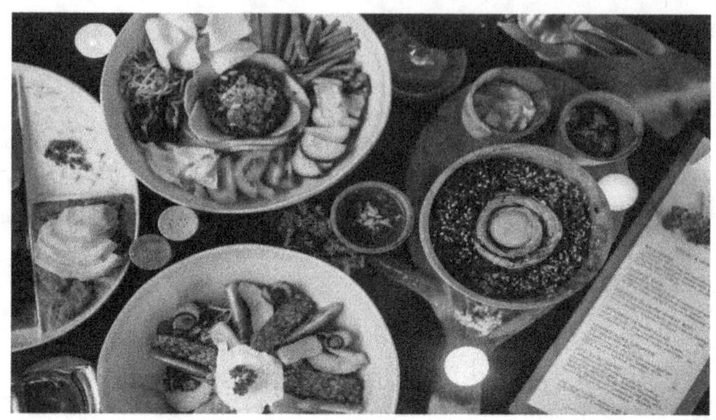

Certainly! Here's a flavorful recipe for Roasted Vegetable and Lentil Salad:

Ingredients:

For Roasted Vegetables:
- 2 cups cherry tomatoes, halved
- 1 zucchini, diced
- 1 red bell pepper, diced
- 1 red onion, sliced
- 2 tablespoons olive oil
- 1 teaspoon dried thyme
- 1 teaspoon dried rosemary
- Salt and black pepper to taste

For Lentils:
- 1 cup dry green or brown lentils
- 3 cups vegetable broth or water
- 1 bay leaf (optional)

- Salt to taste

For Salad:
- Roasted vegetables
- Cooked lentils
- 1/4 cup fresh parsley, chopped
- 1/4 cup feta cheese, crumbled (optional)

For Dressing:
- 3 tablespoons olive oil
- 2 tablespoons balsamic vinegar
- 1 teaspoon Dijon mustard
- 1 clove garlic, minced
- Salt and black pepper to taste

Instructions:

For Roasted Vegetables:

Preheat Oven:
  - Assign 200°C, or 400°F, as the oven temperature.

Prepare Vegetables:
  - In a large bowl, toss halved cherry tomatoes, diced zucchini, diced red bell pepper, and sliced red onion with olive oil, dried thyme, dried rosemary, salt, and black pepper.

Roast Vegetables:
  - Place the vegetables on a baking sheet in a single layer. Roast the vegetables for 20 to 25

minutes, or until they are soft and have begun to caramelize, in a preheated oven.

For Lentils:

Rinse and Cook Lentils:
   - Rinse the lentils under cold water. In a saucepan, combine lentils, vegetable broth or water, and a bay leaf if using. Bring to a boil, then reduce heat to low, cover, and simmer for about 20-25 minutes or until lentils are tender. Drain any excess liquid and remove the bay leaf. Season with salt.

For Salad:

Assemble Salad:
   - In a large bowl, combine the roasted vegetables, cooked lentils, chopped fresh parsley, and crumbled feta cheese if using.

For Dressing:

 Prepare Dressing:
   - In a small bowl, whisk together olive oil, balsamic vinegar, Dijon mustard, minced garlic, salt, and black pepper.

Drizzle Dressing:
   - After drizzling the salad with dressing, toss everything until thoroughly coated.

Serve:
   - Serve the Roasted Vegetable and Lentil Salad
at room temperature or chilled, and enjoy your
wholesome and flavorful meal!

This salad is not only hearty and nutritious but also
a great combination of roasted vegetables and
protein-rich lentils. Feel free to adjust the
ingredients or add your favorite herbs for extra
freshness.

3. Butternut Squash and Apple Soup:

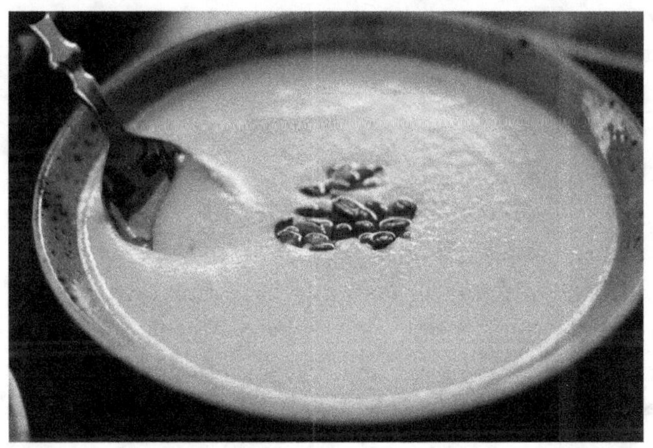

Certainly! Here's a comforting recipe for Butternut
Squash and Apple Soup:

Ingredients:

- One medium butternut squash that has been chopped, skinned, and seeded
- 2 apples, peeled, cored, and diced (use sweet varieties like Gala or Honeycrisp)
- 1 onion, chopped
- 2 carrots, peeled and chopped
- 2 cloves garlic, minced
- 1 teaspoon fresh ginger, grated
- 4 cups vegetable broth
- 1 teaspoon curry powder
- 1/2 teaspoon ground cinnamon
- 1/4 teaspoon nutmeg
- Salt and black pepper to taste
- 2 tablespoons olive oil
- One cup of optional coconut milk (for creaminess)
- Fresh chives or parsley for garnish (optional)

Instructions:

Sauté Vegetables:
   - Warm up the olive oil in a big pot over medium heat. Add chopped onion, carrots, garlic, and grated ginger. Sauté until the vegetables are softened.

Add Squash and Apples:
   - Add apples and cubed butternut squash to the saucepan. Continue to cook for another 5 minutes, stirring occasionally.

Season:

- Sprinkle curry powder, ground cinnamon, nutmeg, salt, and black pepper over the vegetables. Stir well to coat.

Pour in Broth:
- Pour in vegetable broth, ensuring that the vegetables are fully submerged. Bring the mixture to a simmer.

Simmer:
- Reduce heat to low, cover the pot, and let the soup simmer for about 20-25 minutes or until the butternut squash is tender.

Blend Soup:
- Puree the soup with an immersion blender until it's smooth. Alternatively, pour the soup into a blender in batches and process until smooth. Be cautious when blending hot liquids.

Optional Coconut Milk:
- If using coconut milk for creaminess, add it to the blended soup and stir until well combined.

Adjust Seasoning:
- Taste the soup and adjust seasoning if needed. Depending on your taste, you can add extra spices, salt, or pepper.

Serve:

   - Ladle the Butternut Squash and Apple Soup into bowls. If preferred, add some parsley or fresh chives as a garnish.

 Enjoy:
   - Enjoy this warming and flavorful Butternut Squash and Apple Soup as a comforting meal!

This soup combines the sweetness of butternut squash and apples with warm spices for a delightful autumn flavor. The optional addition of coconut milk adds a creamy texture. Feel free to customize the spices or consistency based on your taste.

These recipes offer a variety of flavors and textures, combining creativity with nutritious ingredients in salads and soups to satisfy your palate and appetite.

CHAPTER FIVE

DINNER FOR HEART WELLNESS

"Dinner for Heart Wellness" refers to a carefully curated selection of meals designed to promote heart health and overall well-being during the evening meal. These dinners are thoughtfully crafted to include ingredients that are known to support cardiovascular health, such as lean proteins, whole grains, heart-healthy fats, and a variety of fruits and vegetables.

The emphasis on heart wellness in dinner choices recognizes the significance of the evening meal in contributing to overall nutritional intake and the potential impact on heart health. The goal is to create delicious and satisfying dinners that not only taste good but also provide essential nutrients to support cardiovascular function and reduce the risk of heart-related issues.

Common components of dinners for heart wellness might include:

1. **Lean Proteins:** Incorporating lean sources of protein, such as poultry, fish, legumes, and tofu, which are low in saturated fats and beneficial for heart health.

2. **Whole Grains:** Choosing whole grains like brown rice, quinoa, or whole wheat pasta to provide fiber and important nutrients that contribute to heart wellness.

3. **Heart-Healthy Fats:** Including sources of unsaturated fats, such as olive oil, avocados, and nuts, which can help lower bad cholesterol levels and support heart health.

4. **Colorful Vegetables:** Including a variety of colorful vegetables to provide antioxidants, vitamins, and minerals that contribute to overall cardiovascular well-being.

5. **Moderation in Sodium:** Being mindful of sodium intake by using herbs, spices, and other flavoring options to season meals instead of excessive salt.

6. **Balanced Meals:** Creating balanced meals that include a combination of protein, carbohydrates, and healthy fats to ensure a well-rounded and satisfying dinner.

7. **Portion Control:** Practicing portion control to avoid overeating and maintain a healthy weight, which is crucial for heart wellness.

By focusing on these principles, "Dinner for Heart Wellness" aims to promote a heart-healthy lifestyle, providing individuals with the tools to make informed and nutritious choices during their evening meals to support long-term cardiovascular health.

FLAVORFUL GAINS AND VEGETABLES ENTRÉES

Certainly! Here are 5 flavorful grain and vegetable entrees, each with detailed instructions:

1. Quinoa-Stuffed Bell Peppers:

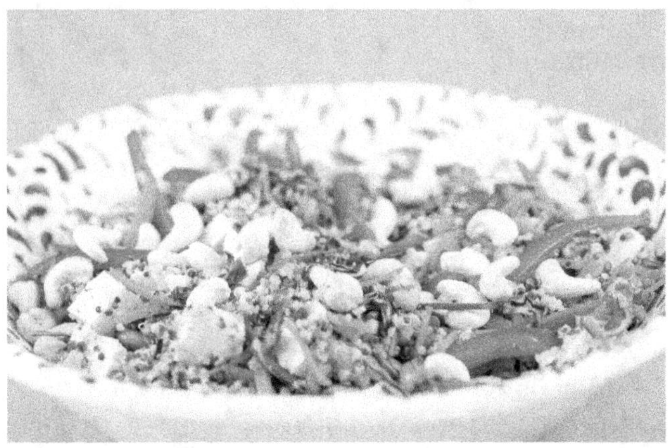

Certainly! This is a tasty recipe for bell peppers stuffed with quinoa:

Ingredients:

- 4 large bell peppers, halved and seeds removed
- 1 cup quinoa, rinsed

- 2 cups vegetable broth or water
- 1 can (15 oz) black beans, drained and rinsed
- One cup of corn kernels, either frozen or fresh
- 1 cup cherry tomatoes, diced
- 1/2 cup red onion, finely chopped
- 2 cloves garlic, minced
- 1 teaspoon ground cumin
- 1 teaspoon chili powder
- Salt and pepper to taste
- 1 cup shredded cheese (cheddar, Monterey Jack, or a blend)
- Fresh cilantro or parsley for garnish (optional)
- Olive oil for drizzling

Instructions:

Preheat Oven:
   - Set the oven temperature to 375°F, or 190°C.

Prepare Quinoa:
   - In a medium saucepan, combine quinoa and vegetable broth (or water). After bringing to a boil, lower the heat to a simmer, cover, and let the quinoa cook for approximately 15 minutes, or until the liquid has been absorbed.

Prepare Bell Peppers:
   - Cut bell peppers in half lengthwise and remove seeds and membranes. Place the pepper halves in a baking dish.

Sauté Vegetables:

- Heat the olive oil in a big skillet over medium heat. Add garlic and red onion, sauté until softened.
   - Add black beans, corn, cherry tomatoes, cumin, chili powder, salt, and pepper. Cook for an additional 3-5 minutes.

 Combine Ingredients:
   - Combine the cooked quinoa with the sautéed vegetable mixture. Mix well.

Stuff Bell Peppers:
   - Spoon the quinoa mixture into each bell pepper half, pressing down gently.
   - Lightly drizzle a little olive oil over the tops.

Bake:
   - Sprinkle shredded cheese over each stuffed pepper.
   - Cover the baking dish with aluminum foil and bake in the preheated oven for 25-30 minutes or until the peppers are tender.

Garnish and Serve:
   - Remove from the oven and garnish with fresh cilantro or parsley if desired.
   - Serve the quinoa-stuffed bell peppers warm.

These quinoa-stuffed bell peppers make for a nutritious and colorful meal. Feel free to customize the recipe by adding your favorite toppings or serving with a side of salsa or guacamole. Enjoy your wholesome and flavorful dish!

2. Eggplant and Chickpea Curry:

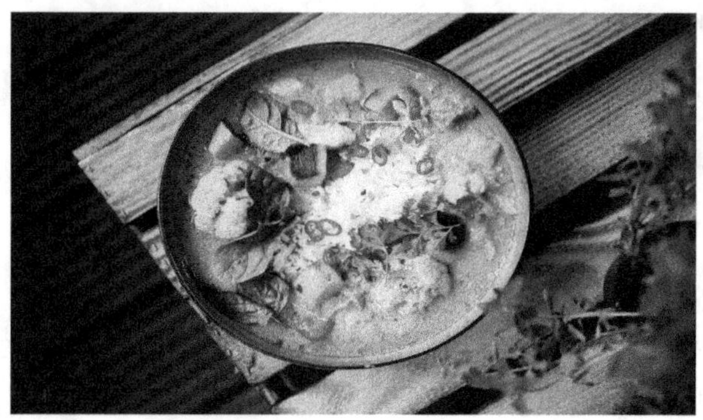

 Certainly! Here's a simple and flavorful recipe for Eggplant and Chickpea Curry:

Ingredients:

- 1 large eggplant, diced
- 1 can (15 oz) chickpeas, drained and rinsed
- 1 onion, finely chopped
- 3 cloves garlic, minced
- 1-inch piece of ginger, grated
- 1 can (14 oz) diced tomatoes
- 1 can (14 oz) coconut milk
- 2 tablespoons curry powder
- 1 teaspoon ground cumin
- 1 teaspoon ground coriander
- 1/2 teaspoon turmeric

- 1/2 teaspoon cayenne pepper (adjust to taste for spice level)
- Salt and pepper to taste
- 2 tablespoons cooking oil
- Fresh cilantro for garnish
- Cooked rice for serving

Instructions:

Preparation:
   - In a big pan, warm up the oil over medium heat.
   - Saute the sliced onions till they become transparent.

Aromatics:
   - Grated ginger and minced garlic should be added to the onions. Add one more minute of sautéing until aromatic.

Spice Mix:
   - Stir in curry powder, ground cumin, ground coriander, turmeric, cayenne pepper, salt, and pepper. Mix well to coat the onions and aromatics with the spices.

Vegetables:
   - Add diced eggplant to the pan and cook until it starts to soften, stirring occasionally.

Chickpeas and Tomatoes:
   - Pour in the drained and rinsed chickpeas, followed by diced tomatoes. Stir to combine.

Simmer:
   - Lower the heat and let the mixture simmer for about 10-15 minutes, allowing the flavors to meld and the eggplant to fully cook.

Coconut Milk:
   - Pour in the coconut milk, stirring well. Simmer for an additional 5-7 minutes until the curry reaches your desired consistency.

Adjust Seasoning:
   - Taste and adjust the seasoning, adding more salt, pepper, or spice as needed.

Garnish and Serve:
   - Remove from heat and garnish with fresh cilantro.

Serve:
   - Serve the Eggplant and Chickpea Curry over cooked rice or your favorite grain.

This Eggplant and Chickpea Curry is not only hearty and satisfying but also packed with rich flavors. Adjust the spice levels according to your preference and enjoy a delicious, plant-based curry!

3. Lemon Garlic Orzo with Roasted Vegetables:

Certainly! Here's a delightful recipe for Lemon Garlic Orzo with Roasted Vegetables:

Ingredients:

- 1 cup orzo pasta
- 2 cups mixed vegetables (such as cherry tomatoes, bell peppers, zucchini, and red onion), diced
- 3 tablespoons olive oil
- 4 cloves garlic, minced
- Zest of 1 lemon
- Juice of 1 lemon
- 1 teaspoon dried oregano
- Salt and pepper to taste
- Fresh parsley for garnish
- Grated Parmesan cheese (optional)

Instructions:

Preheat Oven:
   - Set the oven temperature to 400°F, or 200°C.

Roast Vegetables:
   - Toss the diced vegetables with 2 tablespoons of olive oil, minced garlic, dried oregano, salt, and pepper.
   - Arrange all of the vegetables on a baking sheet in a single layer.
   - Roast for 20 to 25 minutes, or until the veggies are soft and starting to caramelize, in a preheated oven.

Cook Orzo:
 - While the vegetables are roasting, cook the orzo according to package instructions. Drain and set aside.

Prepare Lemon Garlic Dressing:
 - In a small bowl, whisk together the remaining 1 tablespoon of olive oil, lemon zest, lemon juice, and a pinch of salt.

Combine Ingredients:
 - In a large bowl, toss the cooked orzo with the roasted vegetables.
 - Pour the lemon garlic dressing over the orzo and vegetables, tossing to coat evenly.

Garnish and Serve:
 - Add some fresh parsley and, if you'd like, some grated Parmesan cheese as garnish.
 - Serve the Lemon Garlic Orzo with Roasted Vegetables warm.

This dish offers a vibrant and refreshing combination of flavors from the lemon, garlic, and roasted vegetables. It's a versatile recipe that can be enjoyed as a light main course or a flavorful side dish. You are welcome to alter the vegetable selection to suit your tastes. Enjoy your Lemon Garlic Orzo with Roasted Vegetables!

4. Lentil and Vegetable Stir-Fry:

Certainly! Here's a tasty recipe for Lentil and Vegetable Stir-Fry:

Ingredients:

- 1 cup dry green or brown lentils, rinsed and cooked
- 2 cups mixed vegetables (broccoli florets, bell peppers, snap peas, carrots), chopped
- 3 tablespoons soy sauce
- 1 tablespoon sesame oil
- 2 tablespoons vegetable oil
- 3 cloves garlic, minced
- 1 tablespoon ginger, grated
- 1 tablespoon rice vinegar
- 1 tablespoon hoisin sauce
- 1 teaspoon honey or maple syrup
- 1 green onion, sliced (for garnish)
- Sesame seeds (for garnish)
- Cooked brown rice or quinoa (for serving)

Instructions:

Cook Lentils:
   - Rinse lentils and cook them according to package instructions until they are tender but still hold their shape.

 Prepare Sauce:

- In a small bowl, whisk together soy sauce, sesame oil, rice vinegar, hoisin sauce, and honey. Set aside.

Stir-Fry Vegetables:
   - Vegetable oil should be heated over medium-high heat in a large wok or skillet.
   - Stir-fry the grated ginger and minced garlic for 30 seconds or until fragrant.
   - Add chopped vegetables to the wok and stir-fry for 5-7 minutes until they are tender-crisp.

Combine Lentils and Sauce:
   - Add the cooked lentils to the wok, and pour the prepared sauce over the vegetables and lentils.
   - Toss everything together until well-coated and heated through.

 Adjust Seasoning:
   - Taste and adjust the seasoning, adding more soy sauce or honey if needed.

Serve:
   - Serve the Lentil and Vegetable Stir-Fry over cooked brown rice or quinoa.

Garnish:
   - Sesame seeds and sliced green onions make a flavorful and textural garnish.

This Lentil and Vegetable Stir-Fry is a nutritious and satisfying dish that provides a good balance of protein and fiber. It's a versatile recipe, so feel free to customize the vegetables based on what you have available. Enjoy your delicious and wholesome stir-fry!

5. Spaghetti Squash Primavera:

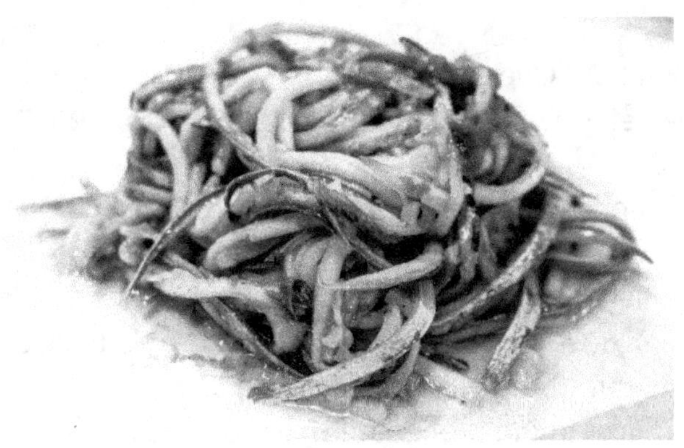

Certainly! Here's a tasty recipe for Spaghetti Squash Primavera:

Ingredients:

- 1 medium-sized spaghetti squash
- 2 tablespoons olive oil
- 3 cloves garlic, minced
- 1 small red onion, thinly sliced
- 1 bell pepper (any color), thinly sliced
- 1 medium zucchini, julienned
- 1 medium carrot, julienned
- 1 cup cherry tomatoes, halved
- 1/2 cup fresh or frozen peas

- Salt and black pepper to taste
- One tspn dry Italian herbs (such basil, thyme, or oregano)
- Grated Parmesan cheese (optional, for serving)
- Fresh basil or parsley for garnish

Instructions:

Preheat Oven:
   - Set the oven temperature to 375°F, or 190°C.

Prepare Spaghetti Squash:
   - Scoop out the seeds after cutting the spaghetti squash in half lengthwise.
   - Squash halves should be placed on a baking pan, cut side down.
   - Bake in the preheated oven for about 40-45 minutes or until the squash is tender.

Scrape Spaghetti Squash:
   - Let the squash cool slightly, then use a fork to scrape the flesh into spaghetti-like strands. Set aside.

 Prepare Vegetables:
   - In a large skillet, the olive oil should be heated over medium heat.
   - Add minced garlic and sliced red onion, sautéing until softened.

 Add Vegetables:

- Add bell pepper, julienned zucchini, julienned carrot, cherry tomatoes, and peas to the skillet.
   - The veggies should be sautéed for 5 to 7 minutes until they are crisp-tender.

Combine with Spaghetti Squash:
   - Add the scraped spaghetti squash strands to the skillet, tossing everything together until well combined.

Season:
   - Season the dish with salt, black pepper, and dried Italian herbs. Adjust the seasoning to taste.

Serve:
   - Serve the Spaghetti Squash Primavera in bowls, garnished with grated Parmesan cheese (if using) and fresh basil or parsley.

This Spaghetti Squash Primavera is a colorful and flavorful alternative to traditional pasta dishes. It's loaded with vibrant vegetables and makes for a delicious, low-carb meal. Enjoy your nutritious and satisfying spaghetti squash creation!

SMART SWAPS FOR HEART-CONSCIOUS COOKING

Certainly! Here are 6 heart-conscious cooking recipes with detailed instructions, featuring smart swaps for healthier options:

1. Cauliflower Pizza Crust:

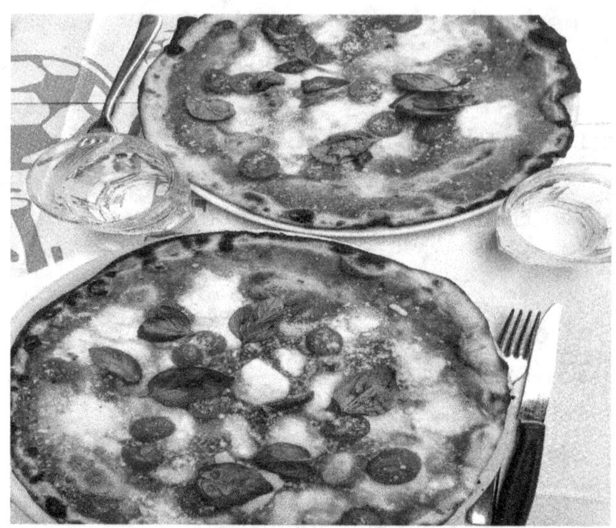

 Certainly! Here's a recipe for Cauliflower Pizza
Crust, a low-carb and gluten-free alternative to
traditional pizza crust:

Ingredients:

- 1 medium-sized cauliflower head
- 1 egg, beaten
- 1 cup shredded mozzarella cheese
- 1 teaspoon dried oregano
- 1 teaspoon dried basil
- 1/2 teaspoon garlic powder
- Salt and black pepper to taste
- Olive oil (for brushing)

Instructions:

Preheat Oven:
   - Preheat your oven to 400°F (200°C). Place a pizza stone or parchment paper on a baking sheet.

Prepare Cauliflower:
   - In a food processor, pulse the chopped cauliflower until it resembles fine crumbs.

Steam Cauliflower:
   - Place the cauliflower crumbs in a microwave-safe bowl and microwave for 4-5 minutes or until softened.
   - Allow the cauliflower to cool slightly.

 Drain Excess Moisture:
   - Transfer the steamed cauliflower to a clean kitchen towel or cheesecloth.
   - Take out as much moisture as possible. This step is crucial for a crisp crust.

Mix Ingredients:
   - In a bowl, combine the cauliflower, beaten egg, shredded mozzarella, oregano, basil, garlic powder, salt, and black pepper. Mix until well combined.

Shape the Crust:
   - Place the cauliflower mixture on the prepared pizza stone or parchment paper.
   - Press the mixture into a thin, even layer, shaping it into a round pizza crust.

Bake First Round:
   - Bake for about 20 minutes, or until the crust is golden brown, in the preheated oven.

Add Toppings:
   - Remove the crust from the oven and add your favorite pizza toppings.

Bake Again:
   - Return the pizza to the oven, and bake it for a further ten to fifteen minutes, or until the cheese is bubbling and melted.

Serve:
   - Once done, let the cauliflower pizza cool for a few minutes before slicing. Serve and enjoy!

This Cauliflower Pizza Crust provides a tasty and healthier alternative for pizza lovers. Customize it with your preferred toppings for a delicious, low-carb pizza experience.

2. Sweet Potato Nachos:

Certainly! Here's a recipe for Sweet Potato Nachos, a nutritious twist on the classic nachos:

Ingredients:

- 2 large sweet potatoes, washed and thinly sliced into rounds

- 2 tablespoons olive oil
- 1 teaspoon ground cumin
- 1 teaspoon paprika
- 1/2 teaspoon garlic powder
- Salt and black pepper to taste
- One cup of cooked and drained black beans
- One cup of shredded Mexican blend or cheddar cheese
- 1/2 cup cherry tomatoes, diced
- 1/4 cup red onion, finely chopped
- 1/4 cup fresh cilantro, chopped
- Jalapeño slices (optional, for some heat)
- For serving, use sour cream or Greek yogurt.
- Guacamole or salsa (optional, for serving)

Instructions:

Preheat Oven:
   - Set the oven's temperature to 425°F (220°C).

Prepare Sweet Potatoes:
   - In a large bowl, toss sweet potato rounds with olive oil, ground cumin, paprika, garlic powder, salt, and black pepper until evenly coated.

Bake Sweet Potatoes:
   - Arrange the seasoned sweet potato rounds in a single layer on a baking sheet lined with parchment paper.
   - Bake in the preheated oven for 20-25 minutes or until the sweet potatoes are golden and crispy.

Assemble Nachos:
   - Remove the sweet potato rounds from the oven and sprinkle black beans and shredded cheese evenly over the top.
   - Put the baking sheet back in the oven and continue baking for another five to seven minutes, or until the cheese is bubbling and melted.

Add Toppings:
   - Once out of the oven, top the sweet potato nachos with diced cherry tomatoes, chopped red onion, fresh cilantro, and jalapeño slices if desired.

Serve:
   - Serve the sweet potato nachos warm with a dollop of Greek yogurt or sour cream on the side.
   - Optionally, serve with guacamole or salsa for added flavor.

These Sweet Potato Nachos are not only delicious but also packed with nutrients. They make for a satisfying and wholesome snack or appetizer. You are welcome to alter the toppings to suit your tastes. Enjoy your healthier take on nachos!

3. Quinoa and Black Bean Stuffed Bell Peppers:

 Absolutely! Here's a delicious recipe for Quinoa and Black Bean Stuffed Bell Peppers:

Ingredients:

- 4 large bell peppers, halved and seeds removed
- 1 cup quinoa, rinsed
- 2 cups vegetable broth or water
- 1 can (15 oz) black beans, drained and rinsed
- One cup of corn kernels, either frozen or fresh
- 1 cup cherry tomatoes, diced
- 1/2 cup red onion, finely chopped
- 2 cloves garlic, minced
- 1 teaspoon ground cumin
- 1 teaspoon chili powder
- 1/2 teaspoon paprika
- Salt and pepper to taste
- One cup of shredded Mexican blend or cheddar cheese
- Fresh cilantro for garnish
- Avocado slices for serving (optional)
- Lime wedges for serving

Instructions:

Preheat Oven:
   - Set the oven temperature to 375°F, or 190°C.

Prepare Quinoa:
   - In a medium saucepan, combine quinoa and vegetable broth (or water). After bringing to a boil, lower the heat to a simmer, cover, and let the quinoa cook for approximately 15 minutes, or until the liquid has been absorbed.

Prepare Bell Peppers:

- Bell peppers cut in half should be put in a baking dish.

Sauté Vegetables:
- Heat the olive oil in a big skillet over medium heat. Add minced garlic and red onion, sautéing until softened.
- Add corn, black beans, cherry tomatoes, ground cumin, chili powder, paprika, salt, and pepper. Cook for an additional 5-7 minutes until the vegetables are tender.

Combine Ingredients:
- Stir the cooked quinoa into the vegetable mixture until well combined.

Stuff Bell Peppers:
- Spoon the quinoa and black bean mixture into each bell pepper half, pressing down gently.

Top with Cheese:
- Sprinkle shredded cheese over each stuffed pepper.

Bake:
- Cover the baking dish with aluminum foil and bake in the preheated oven for 25-30 minutes or until the peppers are tender.

Garnish and Serve:

- Remove from the oven, garnish with fresh cilantro, and serve the stuffed bell peppers with optional avocado slices and lime wedges.

These Quinoa and Black Bean Stuffed Bell Peppers make for a wholesome and satisfying meal. They're rich in protein, fiber, and flavor. Customize the recipe with your favorite toppings and enjoy a nutritious dish!

4. Cherry tomatoes with pesto-topped zucchini noodles::**

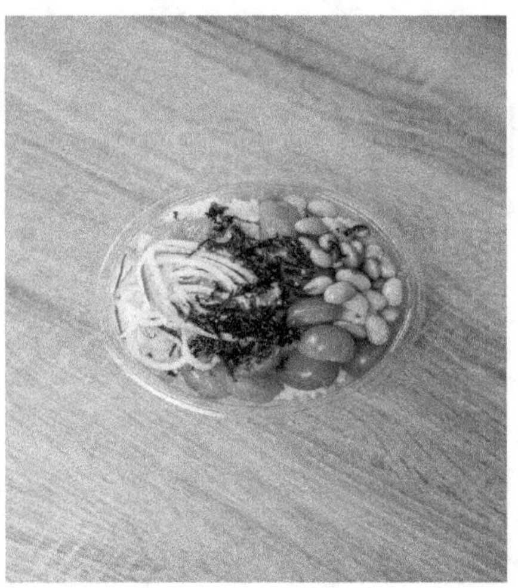

Certainly! Here's a simple and flavorful recipe for Cherry Tomatoes with Pesto-Topped Zucchini Noodles:

Ingredients:

- 2 medium-sized zucchini, spiralized into noodles
- 1 cup cherry tomatoes, halved
- 2 tablespoons pesto sauce (store-bought or homemade)
- 2 tablespoons grated Parmesan cheese (optional)
- Salt and black pepper to taste
- Red pepper flakes that have been crushed (optional; adds heat)
- Fresh basil leaves for garnish

Instructions:

Prepare Zucchini Noodles:
   - Using a spiralizer, create zucchini noodles. If you don't have a spiralizer, you can use a vegetable peeler to make ribbon-like noodles.

Sauté Zucchini Noodles:
   - Heat a large skillet over medium heat. Add a drizzle of olive oil.
   - Add zucchini noodles to the skillet and sauté for 2-3 minutes, or until just tender. Be careful not to overcook; you want the noodles to retain a bit of crunch.

Combine with Cherry Tomatoes:
   - Add halved cherry tomatoes to the skillet with the zucchini noodles. Toss everything together until the tomatoes are slightly softened but still have a fresh crunch.

Add Pesto Sauce:
   - Spoon pesto sauce over the zucchini noodles and cherry tomatoes. Toss well to coat evenly.

Season:
   - Season with salt and black pepper to taste. If you like a bit of heat, you can also add crushed red pepper flakes.

Serve:
   - Transfer the zucchini noodle mixture to a serving plate.
   - Optionally, sprinkle grated Parmesan cheese on top for added flavor.

Garnish:
   - Add some freshly chopped basil as a garnish for a punch of herbaceous freshness.

Enjoy:
   - Serve immediately and enjoy your Cherry Tomatoes with Pesto-Topped Zucchini Noodles!

This dish is a light and vibrant option that's not only delicious but also low in carbs. The combination of fresh cherry tomatoes, zucchini noodles, and flavorful pesto creates a delightful and satisfying meal. Feel free to customize it by adding grilled chicken or shrimp for added protein.

5. Turkey and Quinoa Stuffed Mushrooms:

Certainly! Here's a delicious recipe for Turkey and Quinoa Stuffed Mushrooms:

Ingredients:

- 20-24 large mushrooms, cleaned and stems removed
- 1 cup cooked quinoa
- 1/2 pound ground turkey
- 1/2 onion, finely chopped
- 2 cloves garlic, minced
- 1/2 cup spinach, chopped
- 1/4 cup feta cheese, crumbled (optional)
- 1 teaspoon dried oregano
- 1 teaspoon dried thyme
- Salt and black pepper to taste
- Olive oil for cooking
- Fresh parsley for garnish

Instructions:

Preheat Oven:
   - Set the oven temperature to 375°F, or 190°C.

Prepare Mushrooms:
   - Remove stems from the mushrooms and set aside. The mushroom caps should be put on a baking pan.

Cook Turkey:
- In a skillet, heat olive oil over medium heat. Add chopped onions and minced garlic, sautéing until softened.
- Once added, sauté the ground turkey until browned. Season with dried oregano, dried thyme, salt, and black pepper.

Add Spinach and Quinoa:
- Stir in chopped spinach and cooked quinoa to the turkey mixture. Cook for an additional 2-3 minutes until the spinach wilts.

Stuff Mushrooms:
- Using a spoon, fill each mushroom cap with the turkey and quinoa mixture. Press down gently to pack the filling.

Bake:
- Bake the mushrooms in the preheated oven for 20 to 25 minutes, or until they are soft.

Optional Cheese Topping:
- If using feta cheese, sprinkle crumbled feta over the stuffed mushrooms during the last 5 minutes of baking.

Garnish and Serve:
- Remove from oven and top with freshly chopped parsley.

Enjoy:

- Serve the Turkey and Quinoa Stuffed
Mushrooms warm as a delicious appetizer or a light
meal.

These stuffed mushrooms are not only savory and
flavorful but also a nutritious option. Feel free to
customize the recipe by adding your favorite herbs
or adjusting the filling ingredients to suit your taste.
Enjoy your tasty and protein-packed stuffed
mushrooms!

**6. Greek Yogurt Chicken Salad Lettuce
Wraps:**

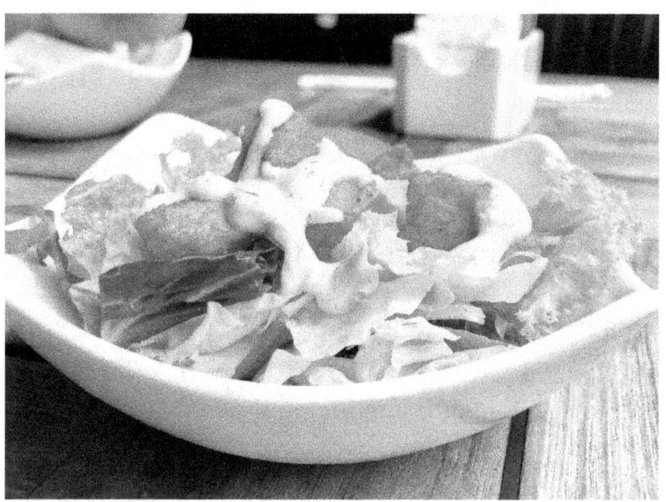

Certainly! Here's a refreshing and healthy recipe
for Greek Yogurt Chicken Salad Lettuce Wraps:

Ingredients:

For Chicken Salad:
- 2 cups cooked chicken breast, shredded or diced
- 1/2 cup Greek yogurt (plain, non-fat)
- 1/4 cup cucumber, finely diced
- 1/4 cup red onion, finely chopped
- 1/4 cup cherry tomatoes, halved
- 1/4 cup Kalamata olives, sliced
- 2 tablespoons feta cheese, crumbled
- 1 tablespoon fresh dill, chopped
- Salt and black pepper to taste

For Lettuce Wraps:
- Big lettuce leaves, like those of butter or iceberg lettuce

Instructions:

Prepare Chicken Salad:
  - In a bowl, combine cooked chicken breast, Greek yogurt, cucumber, red onion, cherry tomatoes, Kalamata olives, feta cheese, and fresh dill.

Season:
  - To taste, add a pinch of salt and black pepper to the chicken salad. Mix well to combine all ingredients.

Assemble Lettuce Wraps:
  - Spoon the Greek Yogurt Chicken Salad onto large lettuce leaves, creating wraps.

Serve:
   - Serve the lettuce wraps immediately, and optionally, garnish with additional fresh dill or a squeeze of lemon juice.

Enjoy:
   - Enjoy these light and flavorful Greek Yogurt Chicken Salad Lettuce Wraps as a healthy and satisfying meal.

These lettuce wraps are a great low-carb and high-protein option, perfect for a light lunch or dinner. The Greek yogurt adds a creamy texture while keeping the dish nutritious. Feel free to customize the recipe by adding your favorite veggies or adjusting the seasonings to suit your taste preferences.

These smart swaps for heart-conscious cooking provide flavorful and nutritious alternatives to traditional recipes, ensuring a heart-healthy approach to your meals.

CHAPTER SIX

SNACKS WITH PURPOSE

Certainly! Here are 4 snacks with purpose recipes, each with detailed instructions:

1. **Almond Butter and Banana Slices:**

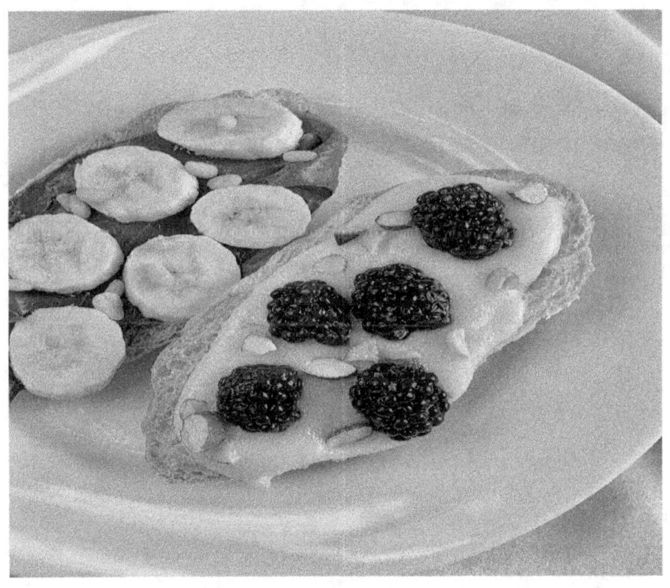

Certainly! Here's a quick and simple recipe for Almond Butter and Banana Slices:

Ingredients:

- 1 ripe banana, peeled and sliced

- 2 tablespoons almond butter
- Optional toppings: Chia seeds, hemp seeds, sliced almonds, or a drizzle of honey

Instructions:

Slice Banana:
- The banana should be peeled and cut into rounds. Depending on your preferences, you can change the slices' thickness.

Spread Almond Butter:
- Take a small spoon and spread almond butter on each banana slice. Ensure an even coating.

Optional Toppings:
- If desired, sprinkle chia seeds, hemp seeds, sliced almonds, or drizzle a bit of honey on top for added flavor and texture.

Serve:
- Arrange the almond butter-covered banana slices on a plate.

Enjoy:
- Enjoy this quick and nutritious snack of Almond Butter and Banana Slices! It's a delightful combination of creamy almond butter and the natural sweetness of bananas.

This snack is not only delicious but also provides a good balance of healthy fats, protein, and carbohydrates. It's perfect for a quick energy boost or a satisfying treat. Feel free to get creative with additional toppings or variations based on your preferences!

2. **Greek Yogurt Parfait:**

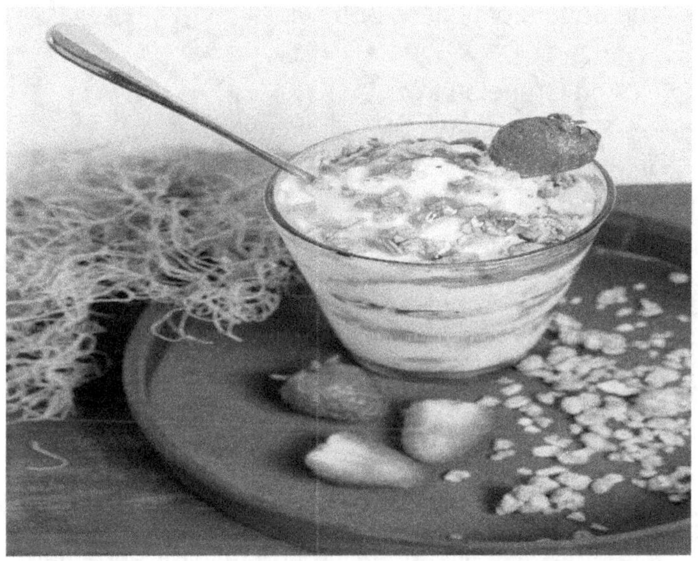

Certainly! Here's a delicious and easy recipe for a Greek Yogurt Parfait:

Ingredients:

- 1 cup Greek yogurt (plain or flavored)
- 1/2 cup granola
- ½ cup of mixed berries, including raspberries, blueberries, and strawberries

- 1 tablespoon honey or maple syrup (optional)
- Nuts or seeds for topping (optional)

Instructions:

Layer Greek Yogurt:
   - Start by spooning a layer of Greek yogurt into the bottom of a glass or bowl.

 Add Granola Layer:
   - Sprinkle a layer of granola over the Greek yogurt. This adds a crunchy texture.

Add Berry Layer:
   - Place a layer of mixed berries on top of the granola. You can mix and match berries for a variety of flavors and colors.

Repeat Layers:
   - Repeat the layers by adding more Greek yogurt, granola, and berries until the glass or bowl is filled. Create a visually appealing and tasty arrangement.

Drizzle with Honey (Optional):
   - If you desire additional sweetness, drizzle honey or maple syrup over the top.

Top with Nuts or Seeds (Optional):
   - For added crunch and nutritional value, sprinkle nuts or seeds on the top layer.

Serve:

- Serve the Greek Yogurt Parfait immediately and enjoy the combination of creamy yogurt, crunchy granola, and sweet berries.

This Greek Yogurt Parfait is not only a delightful treat but also a nutritious option packed with protein, fiber, and antioxidants from the berries. Feel free to customize it with your favorite fruits, nuts, or seeds for a personalized touch!

3. **Hummus and Veggie Sticks:**

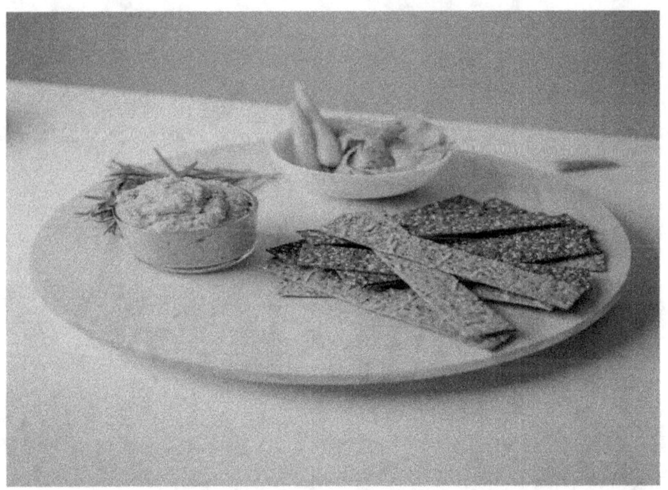

Certainly! Here's a simple and healthy recipe for Hummus and Veggie Sticks:

Ingredients:

- 1 cup hummus (store-bought or homemade)

- Assorted vegetable sticks for dipping:
  - Carrot sticks
  - Cucumber slices
  - Bell pepper strips (assorted colors)
  - Celery sticks
  - Cherry tomatoes

Instructions:

Prepare Vegetables:
  - Wash and cut assorted vegetables into sticks or slices suitable for dipping.

Serve Hummus:
  - Spoon the hummus into a bowl or place it in the center of a serving plate.

 Arrange Vegetable Sticks:
  - Arrange the vegetable sticks around the hummus bowl or plate, creating a colorful and appetizing display.

Dip and Enjoy:
  - Dip the vegetable sticks into the hummus and enjoy this nutritious and satisfying snack.

Variations:
  - You are welcome to alter the vegetable selection to suit your tastes. You can also add additional items like cherry tomatoes or radishes.

This Hummus and Veggie Sticks snack is not only delicious but also provides a good balance of protein, healthy fats, and vitamins from the colorful array of vegetables. It's perfect for a quick and nutritious appetizer or snack.

4. **Trail Mix with Nuts and Seeds:**

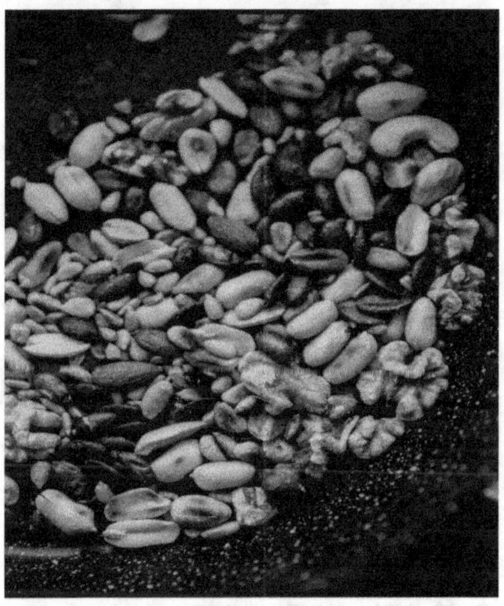

Certainly! Here's a simple recipe for a homemade Trail Mix with Nuts and Seeds:

Ingredients:

- 1 cup almonds
- 1 cup walnuts
- 1/2 cup pumpkin seeds (pepitas)
- 1/2 cup sunflower seeds

- 1/2 cup cashews
- 1/2 cup dried cranberries or raisins
- 1/4 cup dark chocolate chips or chunks
- 1/4 cup unsweetened coconut flakes (optional)
- 1 teaspoon cinnamon (optional)
- Pinch of salt

Instructions:

Preheat Oven (Optional):
   - Preheat your oven to 350°F (175°C) if you want to toast the nuts and seeds for added flavor.

 Toast Nuts and Seeds (Optional):
   - Spread almonds, walnuts, pumpkin seeds, sunflower seeds, and cashews on a baking sheet. Toast in the preheated oven for about 8-10 minutes, stirring halfway through. Watch carefully to avoid burning.

 Combine Ingredients:
   - In a large bowl, combine the toasted or raw nuts and seeds. Add dried cranberries or raisins, dark chocolate chips or chunks, unsweetened coconut flakes (if using), cinnamon (if using), and a pinch of salt.

Mix Well:
   - Toss all the ingredients together until well mixed. Ensure an even distribution of nuts, seeds, and dried fruits.

Store:
   - Transfer the trail mix to an airtight container for storage.

 Enjoy:
   - Enjoy your homemade Trail Mix with Nuts and Seeds as a convenient and energy-boosting snack!

This trail mix is not only delicious but also a great source of healthy fats, protein, and a variety of nutrients. Feel free to customize the mix by adding your favorite nuts, seeds, or dried fruits. It's perfect for on-the-go snacking or as a topping for yogurt or oatmeal.

These snacks with purpose are not only delicious but also provide a combination of nutrients to keep you fueled and satisfied throughout the day.

NOURISHING NIBBLES FOR ANYTIME

Certainly! Here are 3 nourishing nibbles recipes with detailed instructions:

1. **Apple Slices with Nut Butter:**

Certainly! Here's a quick and tasty recipe for Apple Slices with Nut Butter:

Ingredients:

- 2 apples (choose your favorite variety)
- 1/4 cup almond butter or peanut butter
- 1 tablespoon honey or maple syrup (optional)
- 1/4 teaspoon ground cinnamon (optional)
- Sliced almonds or crushed walnuts for topping (optional)

Instructions:

Prepare Apples:
  - Wash the apples and slice them into thin rounds or wedges. You can also remove the core if preferred.

Spread Nut Butter:
  - Take a small spoon and spread almond butter or peanut butter on each apple slice.

 Optional Sweetener:
  - If desired, drizzle honey or maple syrup over the nut butter for added sweetness.

Optional Cinnamon:
  - Sprinkle a little ground cinnamon over the apple slices for extra flavor.

Top with Nuts (Optional):
  - For added crunch, top the nut butter-covered apple slices with sliced almonds or crushed walnuts.

Serve:
   - Arrange the Apple Slices with Nut Butter on a plate or serving tray.

Enjoy:
   - Enjoy this delicious and nutritious snack that combines the natural sweetness of apples with the richness of nut butter.

This snack is not only satisfying but also provides a good balance of fiber, healthy fats, and natural sugars. It's a quick and wholesome option for a snack or light dessert. Feel free to experiment with different nut butters or toppings based on your preferences!

2. **Chia Pudding Parfait:**

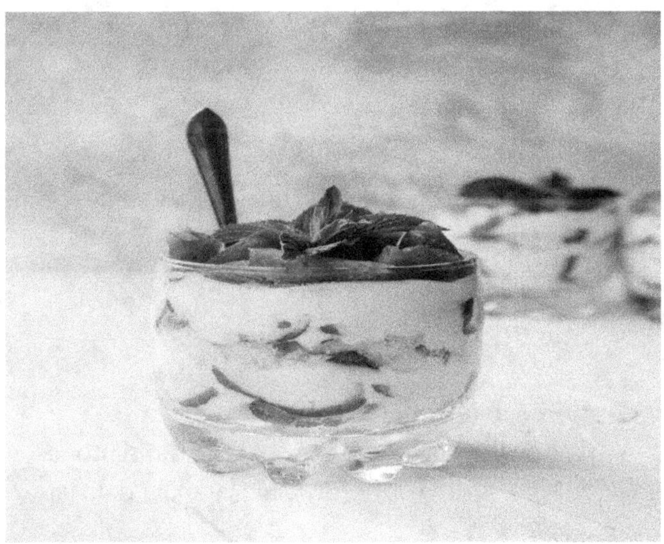

Certainly! Here's a delightful recipe for a Chia Pudding Parfait:

Ingredients:

For Chia Pudding:

- 1/4 cup chia seeds
- One cup almond milk, or any other type of milk you prefer
- 1 tablespoon maple syrup or honey
- 1/2 teaspoon vanilla extract

For Parfait Assembly:

- 1 cup Greek yogurt
- Fresh berries (strawberries, blueberries, raspberries)
- Granola
- Honey for drizzling (optional)

Instructions:

For Chia Pudding:

Prepare Chia Mixture:
   - In a bowl, whisk together chia seeds, almond milk, maple syrup (or honey), and vanilla extract.

Refrigerate:
   - Cover the bowl and refrigerate the chia mixture
for at least 4 hours or overnight, allowing it to
thicken.

Stir Before Serving:
   - Before assembling the parfait, give the chia
pudding a good stir to ensure an even consistency.

For Parfait Assembly:

 Layer Greek Yogurt:
   - Start by spooning a layer of Greek yogurt into
the bottom of a glass or bowl.

Add Chia Pudding Layer:
   - Spoon a layer of the prepared chia pudding on
top of the Greek yogurt layer.

Layer Fresh Berries:
   - Add a layer of fresh berries on top of the chia
pudding. You can mix and match berries for a
variety of flavors and colors.

Repeat Layers:
   - Repeat the layers by adding more Greek yogurt,
chia pudding, and berries until the glass or bowl is
filled. Create a visually appealing and tasty
arrangement.

Top with Granola:

- Sprinkle granola on the top layer for added crunch and texture.

Optional Honey Drizzle:
- If desired, drizzle a bit of honey on top for extra sweetness.

Serve:
- Serve the Chia Pudding Parfait immediately and enjoy the delightful combination of creamy yogurt, chia pudding, fresh berries, and granola.

This parfait is not only visually appealing but also a nutritious and satisfying breakfast or snack. It's rich in fiber, omega-3 fatty acids from chia seeds, and provides a good balance of flavors and textures. Feel free to customize it with your favorite fruits or toppings!

3. **Edamame Guacamole:**

Certainly! Here's a unique and delicious recipe for Edamame Guacamole:

Ingredients:

- 1 cup shelled edamame, cooked and cooled
- 2 ripe avocados, peeled and pitted
- 1/4 cup red onion, finely chopped
- 1 clove garlic, minced
- 1 medium tomato, diced
- 1/4 cup fresh cilantro, chopped

- Juice of 1 lime
- Salt and black pepper to taste
- Optional: Jalapeño, finely chopped, for added heat

Instructions:

Prepare Edamame:
   - Follow the cooking directions on the package for the shelled edamame. Once cooked, drain and let them cool to room temperature.

Mash Avocados:
   - In a bowl, mash the ripe avocados using a fork or potato masher until you reach your desired level of smoothness.

Combine Ingredients:
   - Add the cooked and cooled edamame, chopped red onion, minced garlic, diced tomato, chopped cilantro, and optional chopped jalapeño to the mashed avocados.

Mix Well:
   - Gently mix all the ingredients until well combined. Be careful not to over-mix to maintain a chunky texture.

Add Lime Juice:
   - Squeeze the juice of one lime into the guacamole and stir to incorporate.

Season:
  - To taste, add more salt and black pepper to the guacamole. Adjust the seasoning according to your preference.

 Chill (Optional):
  - For enhanced flavors, refrigerate the guacamole for about 30 minutes before serving.

 Serve:
  - Serve the Edamame Guacamole with tortilla chips, vegetable sticks, or as a topping for tacos.

This Edamame Guacamole offers a unique twist to the classic guacamole by incorporating the nutty flavor and vibrant color of edamame. It's a nutritious and flavorful dip that's perfect for gatherings or as a healthy snack.

These nourishing nibbles are not only tasty but also provide a mix of essential nutrients, making them ideal for anytime snacking.

MINDFUL PORTION CONTROL

Mindful portion control is a key aspect of maintaining a healthy and balanced diet. It involves being aware of the quantity of food you consume, making intentional choices, and listening to your body's hunger and fullness cues. Here are some tips for practicing mindful portion control:

1. **Use Smaller Plates:**
   - Choose smaller plates to naturally reduce portion sizes and create a visual cue of a full plate.

2. **Fill Half Your Plate with Vegetables:**
   - Load up on non-starchy vegetables to increase the volume of your meal without significantly increasing calories.

3. **Listen to Hunger Cues:**
   - Observe the cues your body gives you about hunger and fullness. Consume food only when you're hungry and quit when you're full.

4. **Slow Down and Chew Thoroughly:**
   - Take your time to eat, savoring each bite. Chewing thoroughly allows your body to recognize fullness more accurately.

5. **Use Your Hand as a Guide:**
   - Your palm can serve as a rough guide for protein portions, your fist for vegetables, a cupped hand for carbs, and your thumb for fats.

6. **Pre-Portion Snacks:**
   - Divide snacks into single servings to avoid mindlessly eating from a larger package.

7. **Be Mindful of Liquid Calories:**

- Pay attention to the caloric content of beverages. Opt for water or herbal tea as low-calorie alternatives to sugary drinks.

8. **Avoid Distractions:**
   - Eat without distractions like TV or computer screens. This allows you to focus on your meal and recognize fullness.

9. **Practice the Plate Method:**
   - Visualize dividing your plate into sections for protein, grains, and vegetables to create a well-balanced meal.

10. **Read Food Labels:**
   - Check serving sizes on food labels to understand the nutritional content and avoid unintentional overeating.

11. **Portion Out Treats:**
   - Enjoy treats in moderation by portioning them out rather than eating directly from the package.

12. **Be Mindful of Emotional Eating:**
   - Identify triggers for emotional eating and find alternative ways to cope with emotions.

13. **Learn to Recognize Satiation:**
   - Pause during your meal to assess if you're satisfied, and avoid eating until you're uncomfortably full.

14. **Plan and Prepare:**
   - Plan meals in advance and prepare appropriately portioned servings to avoid overeating.

15. **Stay Hydrated:**
   - Drink water throughout the day, as dehydration can sometimes be mistaken for hunger.

16. **Practice Gratitude:**
   - Appreciate the flavors, textures, and nourishment in each bite, fostering a positive relationship with food.

By incorporating these mindful portion control practices into your eating habits, you can promote a healthier relationship with food, support weight management, and contribute to overall well-being.

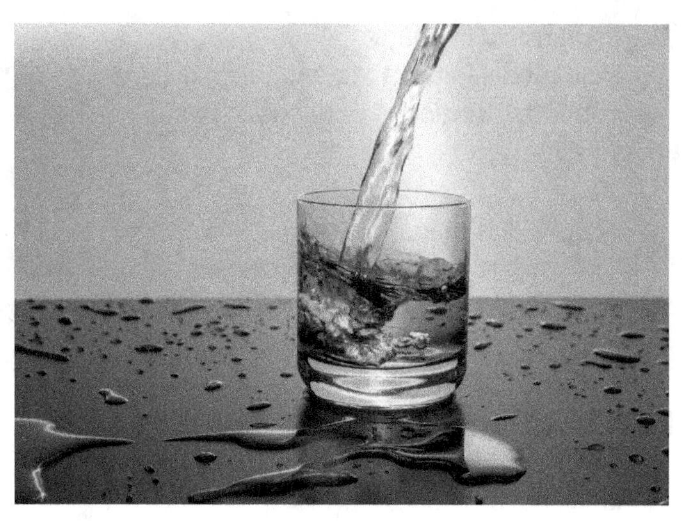

CHAPTER SEVEN

DESSERTS WITH A HEARTFUL TWIST

Certainly! Here are 4 dessert recipes with a heartful twist, each with detailed instructions:

1. **Avocado Chocolate Mousse:**

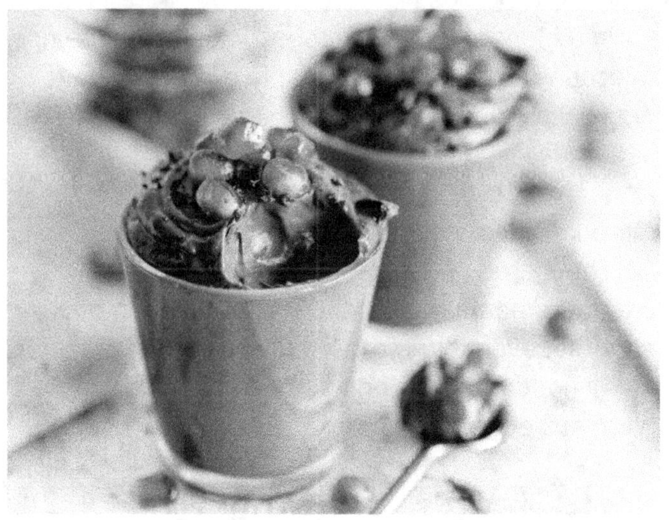

Certainly! Here's a simple and indulgent recipe for Avocado Chocolate Mousse:

Ingredients:

- 2 ripe avocados, peeled and pitted

- 1/4 cup cocoa powder (unsweetened)
- 1/4 cup of either agave nectar or maple syrup
- 1/4 cup almond milk, or any other kind of milk that you like
- 1 teaspoon vanilla extract
- Pinch of salt
- Optional toppings: Fresh berries, sliced almonds, or whipped coconut cream

Instructions:

Blend Avocados:
  - In a blender or food processor, combine the ripe avocados, cocoa powder, maple syrup (or agave nectar), almond milk, vanilla extract, and a pinch of salt.

Blend Until Smooth:
  - The ingredients should be blended until a creamy, smooth consistency is reached. To make sure that everything is thoroughly combined, you might need to pause and scrape down the blender's edges.

Adjust Sweetness:
  - Taste the chocolate mousse and adjust the sweetness by adding more maple syrup or agave nectar if desired.

Chill (Optional):
  - For a firmer texture, you can refrigerate the chocolate mousse for about 1-2 hours.

Serve:
   - Spoon the Avocado Chocolate Mousse into serving bowls or glasses.

 Add Toppings:
   - Garnish with your favorite toppings such as fresh berries, sliced almonds, or a dollop of whipped coconut cream.

Enjoy:
   - Enjoy this rich and creamy Avocado Chocolate Mousse as a delicious and healthier alternative to traditional chocolate mousse.

This dessert is not only decadent but also benefits from the creamy texture of avocados while being naturally sweetened. It's a great way to satisfy chocolate cravings with a nutritious twist!

2. **Whole Wheat Banana Nut Muffins:**

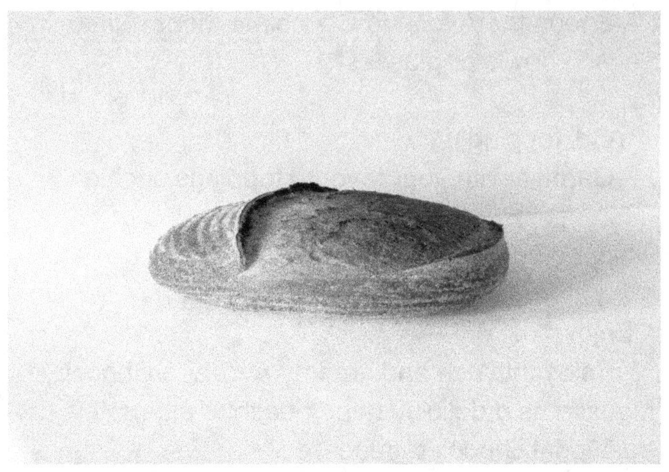

Certainly! Here's a wholesome recipe for Whole Wheat Banana Nut Muffins:

Ingredients:

- 1 1/2 cups whole wheat flour
- 1 teaspoon baking soda
- 1/2 teaspoon baking powder
- 1/4 teaspoon salt
- 3 ripe bananas, mashed
- 1/2 cup honey or maple syrup
- 1/4 cup unsweetened applesauce
- 1 large egg
- 1 teaspoon vanilla extract
- 1/2 cup chopped nuts (walnuts or pecans), plus extra for topping (optional)

Instructions:

Preheat Oven:
   - Set the oven temperature to 350°F (175°C)
.Grease a muffin tray gently or line it with paper
liners.

Mix Dry Ingredients:
   - In a large bowl, whisk together whole wheat
flour, baking soda, baking powder, and salt.

Mash Bananas:
   - In another bowl, mash the ripe bananas with a
fork or potato masher until smooth.

Combine Wet Ingredients:
   - To the mashed bananas, add honey or maple
syrup, unsweetened applesauce, egg, and vanilla
extract. Mix until well combined.

Combine Wet and Dry Mixtures:
   - Mixing until just blended, add the wet
ingredients to the dry components. Do not overmix.

Add Nuts:
   - Gently fold in the chopped nuts into the batter.

 Fill Muffin Cups:
   - Pour the mixture into the muffin tins, filling each
to about two thirds of the way.

 Optional Topping:

- If desired, sprinkle additional chopped nuts on top of each muffin.

Bake:
   - Bake for 18 to 20 minutes, or until a toothpick inserted in the center comes out clean, in a preheated oven.

 Cool:
   - After letting the muffins cool in the pan for a few minutes, move them to a wire rack to finish cooling.

Enjoy:
   - Enjoy these Whole Wheat Banana Nut Muffins as a wholesome and delicious breakfast or snack!

These muffins are a nutritious option, combining the goodness of whole wheat flour, ripe bananas, and nuts. They are perfect for a quick and satisfying bite on busy mornings or as a wholesome treat throughout the day.

3. **Berry and Oat Crumble Bars:**

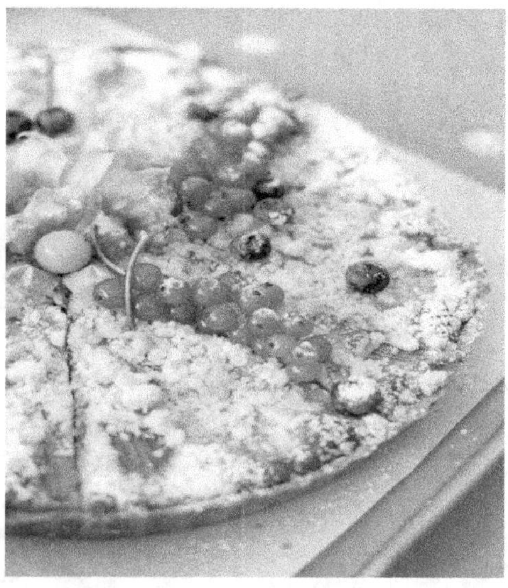

Certainly! Here's a delightful recipe for Berry and Oat Crumble Bars:

Ingredients:

For the Berry Filling:

- Two cups of mixed berries, comprising raspberries, blueberries, and strawberries
- 1/4 cup granulated sugar
- 2 tablespoons lemon juice
- 1 tablespoon cornstarch

For the Oat Crumble:

- 1 1/2 cups old-fashioned oats
- 1 cup whole wheat flour
- 1/2 cup brown sugar, packed
- 1/2 teaspoon baking soda
- 1/4 teaspoon salt
- 1/2 cup unsalted butter, melted
- 1 teaspoon vanilla extract

Instructions:

For the Berry Filling:

Preheat Oven:
  - Preheat your oven to 350°F (175°C). Grease or line a baking pan with parchment paper.

Prepare Berry Mixture:
  - In a bowl, combine mixed berries, granulated sugar, lemon juice, and cornstarch. Toss until the berries are coated evenly.

For the Oat Crumble:

Mix Dry Ingredients:
  - In a separate bowl, mix together old-fashioned oats, whole wheat flour, brown sugar, baking soda, and salt.

Add Wet Ingredients:
  - Add vanilla essence and melted butter to the dry ingredients. Mix until the mixture resembles coarse crumbs.

Assembling and Baking:

Layer Half of the Oat Mixture:
   - Press half of the oat crumble mixture into the bottom of the prepared baking pan to form a firm layer.

Spread Berry Filling:
   - Spread the prepared berry filling over the oat layer in the baking pan.

 Top with Remaining Oat Mixture:
   - Sprinkle the remaining oat crumble mixture evenly over the berry filling.

Bake:
   - Bake in the preheated oven for 30-35 minutes or until the top is golden brown and the berries are bubbly.

Cool:
   - Before slicing the bars into squares, let them cool fully in the pan.

Serve:
   - Serve these delicious Berry and Oat Crumble Bars as a delightful snack or dessert.

These bars are a perfect combination of sweet and tart flavors, with the wholesome goodness of oats and mixed berries. Savour them as a treat together with a cup of coffee or tea!

4. **Coconut and Mango Chia Seed Popsicles:**

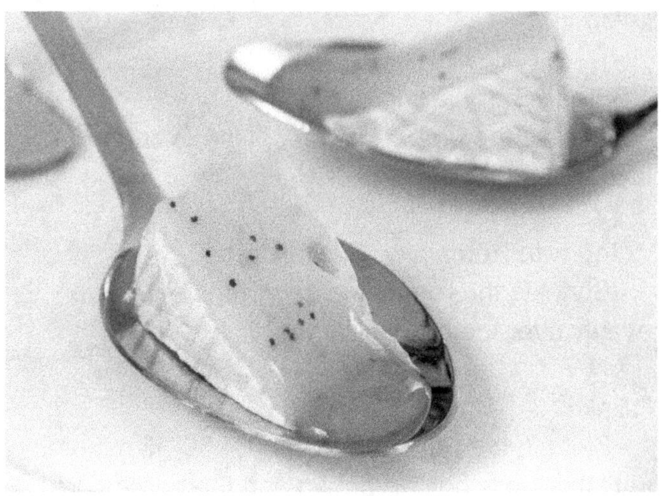

Certainly! Here's a refreshing recipe for Coconut and Mango Chia Seed Popsicles:

Ingredients:

- 1 cup ripe mango, peeled and diced
- 1 can (13.5 oz) coconut milk
- 2 tablespoons chia seeds
- Two to three teaspoons of maple syrup or honey (adjust to taste)
- 1 teaspoon vanilla extract
- Popsicle molds and sticks

Instructions:

Prepare Chia Gel:
   - In a small bowl, mix chia seeds with about 1/4 cup of coconut milk. Allow it to sit for 10-15 minutes, stirring occasionally until it forms a gel-like consistency.

Blend Mango:
   - In a blender, puree the ripe mango until smooth.

Mix Coconut Milk Base:
   - In a separate bowl, combine the remaining coconut milk, honey or maple syrup, and vanilla extract. Mix well.

Combine Coconut Milk Base and Mango Puree:
   - Pour the coconut milk base into the mango puree and stir until well combined.

Add Chia Gel:
   - Add the chia gel to the coconut-mango mixture and stir thoroughly.

Fill Popsicle Molds:
   - Leaving a small amount of space at the top for expansion, pour the mixture into the popsicle molds.

Insert Sticks:

- Place popsicle sticks into the molds. If your molds have lids, make sure they are tightened.

Freeze:
   - Freeze the popsicles for at least 4-6 hours, or until fully set.

 Unmold and Enjoy:
   - Once frozen, run the molds under warm water for a few seconds to help release the popsicles. Gently unmold and enjoy your Coconut and Mango Chia Seed Popsicles!

These popsicles are a delightful combination of tropical flavors and the added nutritional goodness of chia seeds. They make for a perfect cool treat on a warm day!

These desserts with a heartful twist bring together nourishing ingredients and delightful flavors, making them a wholesome treat for any occasion. Enjoy them guilt-free as part of a balanced diet.

SWEET TREATS WITH COMPROMISING HEALTH

Certainly! Here are 3 sweet treats recipes that don't compromise on health, each with detailed instructions:

1. **No-Bake Energy Bites:**

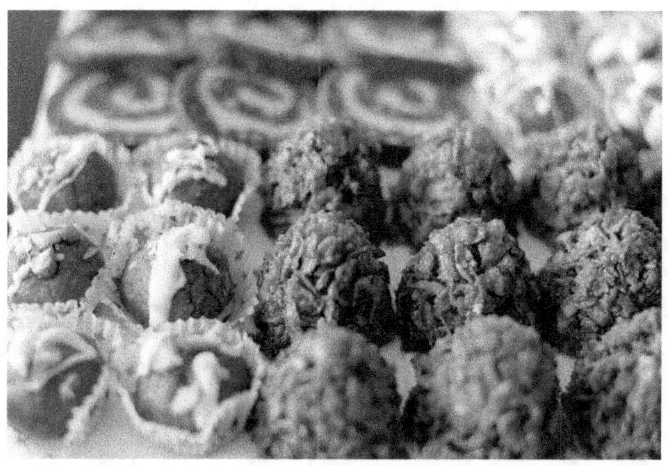

Certainly! Here's a simple recipe for No-Bake Energy Bites:

Ingredients:

- 1 cup old-fashioned oats
- 1/2 cup nut butter (peanut butter, almond butter, or your choice)
- 1/3 cup honey or maple syrup
- 1 cup coconut flakes (unsweetened)
- 1/2 cup ground flaxseed
- 1/2 cup mini chocolate chips
- 1 teaspoon vanilla extract
- A pinch of salt (optional)

Instructions:

Combine Dry Ingredients:
   - In a large bowl, combine oats, coconut flakes, ground flaxseed, mini chocolate chips, and a pinch of salt if desired.

Add Wet Ingredients:
   - Add nut butter, honey or maple syrup, and vanilla extract to the dry ingredients.

 Mix Thoroughly:
   - Stir all the ingredients until well combined. You may need to use your hands to ensure an even mixture.

Chill Dough (Optional):
   - If the mixture is too sticky to handle, you can refrigerate it for about 30 minutes to make it easier to shape.

Shape into Bites:
   - Using your hands, roll little parts of the mixture into bite-sized balls.

 Set:
   - Transfer the energy bites to a plate or tray coated with parchment paper.

Chill:
   - Chill the energy bites in the refrigerator for at least 1 hour to firm up.

Store:

- Once firm, transfer the No-Bake Energy Bites to an airtight container and store in the refrigerator.

Enjoy:
- Enjoy these energy bites as a quick and nutritious snack on the go!

These No-Bake Energy Bites are not only delicious but also packed with fiber, healthy fats, and energy-boosting ingredients. Feel free to customize the recipe by adding your favorite nuts, seeds, or dried fruits. They are ideal for those hectic days when you need a little pick-me-up!

2. **Greek Yogurt and Berry Popsicles:**

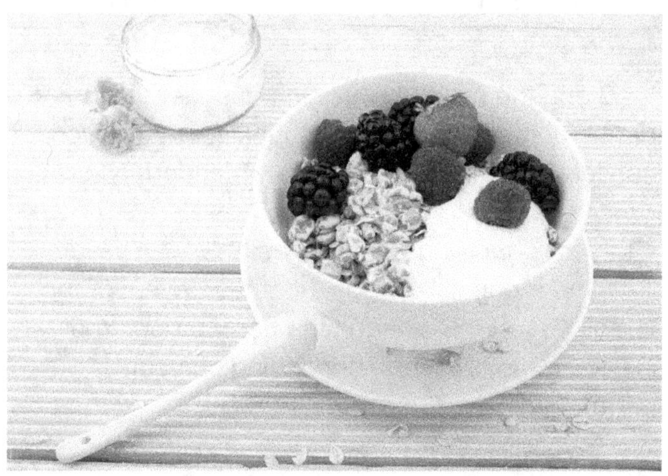

Certainly! Here's a simple and refreshing recipe for Greek Yogurt and Berry Popsicles:

Ingredients:

- 1 cup Greek yogurt
- One cup of mixed berries, including raspberries, blueberries, and strawberries
- Two to three teaspoons of maple syrup or honey (adjust to taste)
- 1 teaspoon vanilla extract (optional)

Instructions:

 Prepare Greek Yogurt Mixture:
  - In a bowl, mix Greek yogurt, honey or maple syrup, and vanilla extract (if using). Stir until well combined.

Blend Berries:
  - Blend the mixed berries in a blender until they are smooth. If you prefer a chunkier texture, you can leave some berries partially blended.

Layer Yogurt and Berry Puree:
  - In your popsicle molds, alternate layers of the Greek yogurt mixture and the berry puree. You can create swirls or layers, depending on your preference.

Insert Sticks:
  - Place popsicle sticks into the molds. If your molds have lids, make sure they are tightened.

Freeze:
   - Freeze the popsicles for at least 4-6 hours, or
until fully set.

Unmold and Enjoy:
   - Once frozen, run the molds under warm water
for a few seconds to help release the popsicles.
Gently unmold and enjoy your Greek Yogurt and
Berry Popsicles!

These popsicles are a delightful combination of
creamy Greek yogurt and the natural sweetness of
mixed berries. They make for a healthy and
delicious frozen treat, perfect for a hot day!

3. **Frozen Banana Bites:**

 Certainly! Here's a simple and healthy recipe for
Frozen Banana Bites:

Ingredients:

- 2 ripe bananas
- 1/4 cup nut butter (peanut butter, almond butter, or
your choice)
- 1/2 cup dark chocolate, melted
- Toppings of your choice (chopped nuts, shredded
coconut, chia seeds, etc.)

Instructions:

Slice Bananas:
  - Peel the ripe bananas and slice them into bite-sized rounds.

Spread Nut Butter:
  - Take each banana slice and spread a thin layer of nut butter on one side.

Create Banana Sandwiches:
  - Create small banana "sandwiches" by placing another banana slice on top, making a little nut butter-filled sandwich.

Freeze:
  - Place the banana bites on a tray lined with parchment paper and freeze for at least 30 minutes or until they are firm.

 Melt Chocolate:
  - Melt the dark chocolate using a double boiler or in the microwave in short intervals, stirring until smooth.

Dip in Chocolate:
  - Dip each frozen banana bite into the melted chocolate, ensuring it is coated evenly. Scrape off any extra chocolate with a fork.

Add Toppings (Optional):

- While the chocolate is still wet, sprinkle your choice of toppings over the banana bites.

Freeze Again:
- Place the chocolate-coated banana bites back on the parchment-lined tray and freeze until the chocolate is set.

Serve:
- Once fully frozen, serve and enjoy these delicious Frozen Banana Bites!

These Frozen Banana Bites make for a delightful and healthier alternative to traditional frozen treats. The combination of creamy banana, nut butter, and dark chocolate creates a satisfying and sweet snack. Feel free to get creative with your favorite toppings!

These sweet treats prioritize health by incorporating nutrient-dense ingredients and minimizing added sugars, providing you with a delicious way to satisfy your sweet cravings.

FRUIT-BASED INDULGENCES AND GUILT-FREE DESSERTS

Certainly! Here are 3 guilt-free fruit-based indulgences and desserts, each with detailed instructions:

1. **Chocolate-Dipped Strawberries:**

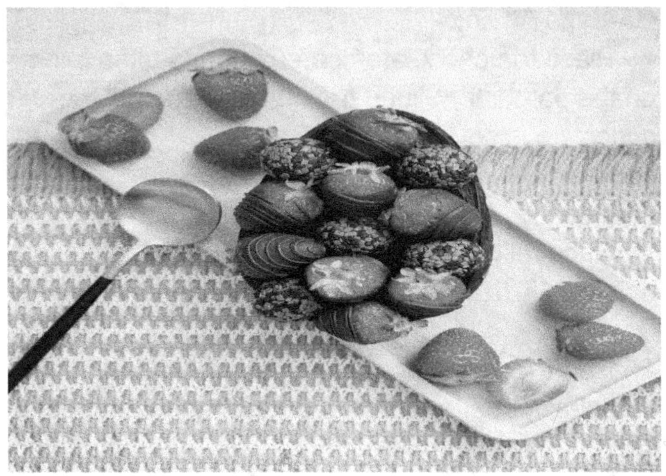

Certainly! Here's a classic and elegant recipe for Chocolate-Dipped Strawberries:

Ingredients:

- Fresh strawberries, washed and dried
- Dark chocolate or semi-sweet chocolate chips
- White chocolate chips (optional for drizzling)
- Toppings of your choice (chopped nuts, shredded coconut, sprinkles, etc.)

Instructions:

Prepare Strawberries:
   - Wash and thoroughly dry the strawberries. For the chocolate to stick to the strawberries properly, they must be totally dry.

Melt Dark Chocolate:
   - In a heatproof bowl, melt the dark chocolate in the microwave or using a double boiler. Stir occasionally until smooth.

Dip Strawberries:
   - Hold each strawberry by the stem and dip it into the melted chocolate, ensuring the strawberry is well-coated. Let any chocolate that's extra fall off.

Place on Parchment Paper:
   - Arrange the strawberries dipped in chocolate onto a parchment paper-lined tray. Verify that they are not in contact with one another.

Optional White Chocolate Drizzle:
   - If desired, melt white chocolate chips and drizzle it over the dark chocolate-coated strawberries using a spoon or a piping bag.

Add Toppings:
   - While the chocolate is still wet, sprinkle your choice of toppings over the strawberries. Common toppings include chopped nuts, shredded coconut, or colorful sprinkles.

Set in the Refrigerator:
   - Place the tray of chocolate-dipped strawberries
in the refrigerator to allow the chocolate to set. This
usually takes about 30 minutes.

Serve and Enjoy:
   - Once the chocolate is fully set, serve and enjoy
these delicious and elegant Chocolate-Dipped
Strawberries!

These Chocolate-Dipped Strawberries are a
delightful treat, perfect for special occasions or as a
sweet indulgence. They can be a wonderful
addition to dessert platters or enjoyed on their own.
Customize them with your favorite toppings for
added flair!

2. **Frozen Banana Pops:**

Certainly! Here's a fun and healthy recipe for
Frozen Banana Pops:

Ingredients:

- Bananas (1 banana makes about 2 pops)
- Yogurt (Greek yogurt or regular yogurt of your
choice)
- Toppings of your choice (chopped nuts, granola,
shredded coconut, mini chocolate chips, etc.)
- Popsicle sticks or sturdy straws

Instructions:

Prepare Bananas:
   - Peel the bananas and cut them in half. Insert a popsicle stick or straw into each banana half, making sure it's sturdy enough to hold the banana.

Dip in Yogurt:
   - Dip each banana half into yogurt, ensuring an even coating. You can use Greek yogurt for a thicker texture or regular yogurt for a lighter option.

Add Toppings:
   - While the yogurt is still wet, roll the banana in your choice of toppings. Get creative and use a variety of toppings for different flavors and textures.

Freeze:
   - Place the banana pops on a tray lined with parchment paper and freeze until solid. This usually takes about 2-3 hours.

Serve and Enjoy:
   - Once frozen, serve these tasty Frozen Banana Pops as a refreshing and nutritious treat!

These Frozen Banana Pops are a great way to enjoy a cool and satisfying snack, especially during warmer weather. They are customizable with various toppings, making them a fun and healthy option for both kids and adults alike.

3. **Watermelon Pizza:**

Certainly! Here's a refreshing and creative recipe for Watermelon Pizza:

Ingredients:

- One circular watermelon slice, about one inch thick
- Greek yogurt or coconut yogurt
- Fresh berries (strawberries, blueberries, raspberries)
- Kiwi slices
- Mint leaves for garnish
- Drizzling with honey or maple syrup is optional.
- Chopped nuts or shredded coconut (optional)

Instructions:

Prepare Watermelon Slice:
  - Cut a round slice from a watermelon, about 1 inch thick, to create the pizza base.

Pat Dry:
  - Pat the watermelon slice dry with a paper towel to remove excess moisture.

Spread Yogurt:
  - Spread a layer of Greek yogurt or coconut yogurt over the watermelon slice, leaving a small border around the edge.

Add Fresh Fruit:
   - Arrange fresh berries, kiwi slices, and any other desired fruits on top of the yogurt-covered watermelon.

 Drizzle with Honey (Optional):
   - For a touch of sweetness, drizzle honey or maple syrup over the fruit-topped watermelon.

 Garnish:
   - Garnish the Watermelon Pizza with mint leaves for a burst of freshness.

Optional Toppings:
   - If desired, sprinkle chopped nuts or shredded coconut over the pizza for added texture.

Slice and Serve:
   - Slice the watermelon pizza into wedges or squares, similar to how you would cut a traditional pizza.

Enjoy:
   - Serve and enjoy this refreshing Watermelon Pizza as a light and hydrating dessert or snack!

This Watermelon Pizza is not only visually appealing but also a healthy and hydrating treat, perfect for summer gatherings or as a fun snack. Feel free to get creative with the fruit toppings based on your preferences!

These guilt-free fruit-based indulgences provide a burst of natural sweetness and essential nutrients, making them a delightful and wholesome choice for dessert.

CHAPTER EIGHT

LIFESTYLE TIPS FOR HEART HEALTH

Maintaining a heart-healthy lifestyle is crucial for overall well-being. Here are lifestyle tips to promote heart health:

1. **Balanced Diet:**
   - Consume a diet rich in fruits, vegetables, whole grains, lean meats, and healthy fats.
   - Limit sodium, added sweets, and fats, both saturated and trans.
   - Be careful of portion sizes and engage in mindful eating.

2. **Regular Exercise:**
   - Aim for 150 minutes or more per week of aerobic activity at a moderate to high level or 75 minutes or more at a high intensity.
   - Make time for strength training activities at least twice a week.
   - Find activities you enjoy to make exercise a regular part of your routine.

3. **Maintain a Healthy Weight:**
   - A balanced diet combined with frequent exercise will help you reach and stay at a healthy weight.

- Consult with healthcare professionals for personalized weight management guidance.

4. **Manage Stress:**
   - Engage in stress-relieving activities like yoga, meditation, deep breathing, or hobbies.
   - Prioritize self-care and ensure adequate sleep to support overall well-being.

5. **Quit Smoking:**
   - If you smoke, get assistance quitting. Smoking is one of the primary risk factors for heart disease.
   - Avoid exposure to secondhand smoke.

6. **Limit Alcohol Consumption:**
   - If you do drink, make sure to do it in moderation. Limit consumption to one drink for women and up to two for males per day.

7. **Regular Health Check-ups:**
   - Make an appointment for routine checkups with your physician to keep an eye on your cholesterol, blood pressure, and general cardiovascular health.
   - Follow recommended screenings for early detection of potential issues.

8. **Stay Hydrated:**
   - Drink an adequate amount of water daily.
   - Limit intake of sugary drinks and excessive caffeinated beverages.

9. **Social Connections:**

- Make sure you have a close social circle of friends and relatives.
   - Engage in activities that bring joy and fulfillment.

10. **Limit Processed Foods:**
   - Reduce intake of processed and packaged foods high in salt, sugar, and unhealthy fats.
   - Choose whole, unprocessed foods whenever possible.

11. **Adequate Sleep:**
   - Every night, try to get seven or nine hours of quality sleep.
   - Create a sleeping-friendly environment and stick to a regular sleep routine.

12. **Hygiene and Health Habits:**
   - Maintain proper hygiene, which includes frequent hand washing, to stop the spread of illnesses.
   - Adhere to recommended vaccinations for overall health.

13. **Educate Yourself:**
   - Stay informed about heart health by reading reputable sources and staying aware of the latest research.
   - Make wise decisions about your well-being and way of life.

Adopting these heart-healthy lifestyle tips can contribute to the prevention of cardiovascular diseases and support overall health. Always consult with healthcare professionals for personalized advice based on your individual health needs.

PHYSICAL ACTIVITY AND ITS ROLES

Physical activity plays a crucial role in maintaining overall health and well-being. Here are some key roles and benefits of regular physical activity:

1. **Cardiovascular Health:**
   - **Role:** Regular exercise strengthens the heart and improves circulation, reducing the risk of heart diseases.
   - **Benefits:** Lower blood pressure, improved cholesterol levels, and enhanced cardiovascular function.

2. **Weight Management:**
   - **Role:** Physical activity helps control body weight by burning calories and increasing metabolism.
   - **Benefits:** Weight maintenance or loss, reduced risk of obesity-related conditions.

3. **Muscle and Bone Health:**
   - **Role:** Weight-bearing and resistance exercises support muscle and bone health.
   - **Benefits:** Increased muscle strength, improved bone density, and reduced risk of osteoporosis.

4. **Mental Health:**
   - **Role:** Exercise releases endorphins, reducing stress, anxiety, and depression.
   - **Benefits:** Enhanced mood, improved cognitive function, and better stress management.

5. **Metabolic Health:**
   - **Role:** Physical activity improves insulin sensitivity and glucose regulation.
   - **Benefits:** Reduced risk of type 2 diabetes and better control of blood sugar levels.

6. **Joint Flexibility and Mobility:**
   - **Role:** Regular movement helps maintain joint flexibility and mobility.
   - **Benefits:** Reduced risk of joint pain, stiffness, and improved overall range of motion.

7. **Improved Sleep:**
   - **Role:** Regular exercise promotes better sleep patterns.
   - **Benefits:** Improved sleep quality and duration, better overall rest and recovery.

8. **Immune System Support:**
   - **Role:** Moderate exercise can boost the immune system.
   - **Benefits:** Reduced susceptibility to illness and quicker recovery.

9. **Cancer Prevention:**

- **Role:** Regular physical activity is associated with a lower risk of certain cancers.
   - **Benefits:** Reduced risk of breast, colon, and other cancers.

10. **Enhanced Respiratory Function:**
   - **Role:** Aerobic exercises improve respiratory function and lung capacity.
   - **Benefits:** Improved breathing efficiency and reduced risk of respiratory issues.

11. **Social Interaction:**
   - **Role:** Group or team activities contribute to social well-being.
   - **Benefits:** Increased social connections, a sense of community, and improved mental health.

12. **Cognitive Function:**
   - **Role:** Physical activity supports cognitive function and brain health.
   - **Benefits:** Improved memory, attention, and reduced risk of cognitive decline.

13. **Longevity:**
   - **Role:** Regular exercise is associated with increased life expectancy.
   - **Benefits:** Enhanced overall quality of life and a longer, healthier lifespan.

14. **Stress Relief:**
   - **Role:** Physical activity acts as a natural stress reliever.

  - **Benefits:** Reduced stress levels, improved ability to cope with daily challenges.

Incorporating a variety of physical activities into your routine, including aerobic, strength, flexibility, and balance exercises, provides comprehensive health benefits. It's important to choose activities that you enjoy to make physical activity a sustainable part of your lifestyle. Always consult with healthcare professionals before starting a new exercise regimen, especially if you have pre-existing health conditions.

STRESS MANAGEMENT TECHNIQUES

Managing stress is crucial for overall well-being. Here are various stress management techniques that can help you cope with and reduce stress:

1. **Deep Breathing:**
   - To trigger the relaxation response in your body, engage in deep breathing exercises.
   - Breathe in slowly through your nose, hold it for a short while, and then release the air through your mouth.

2. **Progressive Muscle Relaxation (PMR):**
   - Systematically tense and then relax different muscle groups to release physical tension.

  - Start from your toes and work your way up to
your head.

3. **Mindfulness Meditation:**
  - To focus attention on the present moment,
practice mindfulness meditation.
  - Focus on your breath, sensations, or a specific
point of focus.

4. **Yoga:**
  - Practice yoga for its combination of physical
postures, breathing, and meditation.
  - Yoga promotes flexibility, strength, and
relaxation.

5. **Guided Imagery:**
  - Use guided imagery to visualize calming and
peaceful scenes.
  - Imagine yourself in a serene environment to
reduce stress and promote relaxation.

6. **Exercise:**
  - Engage in regular physical activity, which
releases endorphins, the body's natural stress
relievers.
  - Choose activities you enjoy, such as walking,
running, or dancing.

7. **Journaling:**
  - Have a notebook handy so you can jot down
your thoughts and feelings.

- Reflecting on your experiences can provide insights and help you process stress.

8. **Time Management:**
  - Set priorities for your projects and divide them into doable chunks.
  - Don't overcommit; instead, set reasonable goals.

9. **Healthy Lifestyle Choices:**
  - Maintain a balanced diet, regular sleep patterns, and stay hydrated.
  - Limit caffeine and alcohol intake, as they can contribute to stress.

10. **Social Support:**
  - Share your feelings with friends, family, or a trusted confidant.
  - Connect with others and build a support network.

11. **Laughter Therapy:**
  - Watch a funny movie, attend a comedy show, or engage in activities that make you laugh.
  - Laughter can trigger the release of endorphins.

12. **Art and Creativity:**
  - Use writing, painting, or other creative mediums to express oneself.
  - Creating art can be a therapeutic endeavor.

13. **Self-Compassion:**

- Treat yourself with kindness and understanding.
- Avoid harsh self-criticism and practice self-compassion.

14. **Cognitive Behavioral Therapy (CBT):**
- Acknowledge and deal with negative thought patterns.
- CBT can help change unhealthy thinking and behavioral patterns.

15. **Nature and Outdoors:**
- Spend time in nature or green spaces.
- Fresh air and natural surroundings can have a calming effect.

16. **Aromatherapy:**
- For relaxation, burn scented candles or use essential oils.
- Aromas with relaxing properties include eucalyptus, lavender, and chamomile.

17. **Limiting Screen Time:**
- Reduce exposure to screens, especially before bedtime.
- Limiting screen time can help with sleep quality.

18. **Listening to Music:**
- Play some calming music or sounds. Music has a strong effect on stress levels and mood.

19. **Volunteering:**
- Take up voluntary work or charitable deeds.

- A sense of contentment and purpose can be obtained via helping others.

20. **Professional Support:**
   - If stress becomes too much for you, get expert help for mental health issues.
   - Therapists can provide coping strategies and support.

Experiment with these techniques to find what works best for you, and consider combining several approaches for a holistic stress management plan. Remember that managing stress is a continual process, and different techniques may be more effective in different situations.

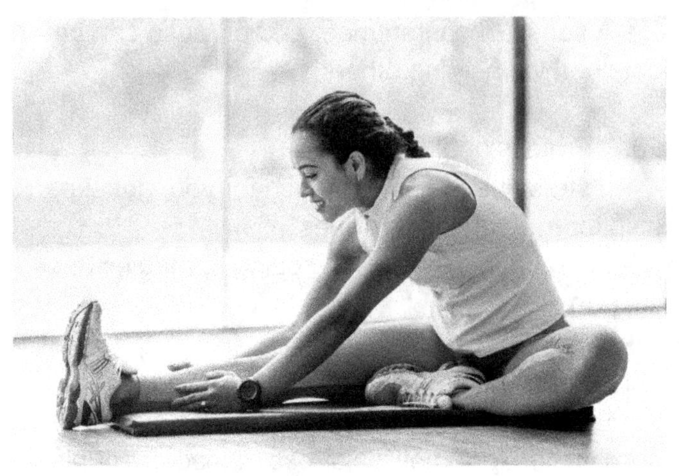

CHAPTER NINE

RECIPES FOR SPECIAL OCCASIONS

Recipes for a special occasion are designed to elevate the dining experience, combining unique flavors, creative presentation, and often a touch of indulgence. Here's an explanation of the key elements involved in crafting recipes for special occasions:

1. **Ingredients Selection:**
   - **Quality Ingredients:** Choose fresh, high-quality ingredients for optimal flavor and texture.
   - **Seasonal and Specialized:** Consider using seasonal produce or specialty items to add uniqueness.

2. **Flavor Balance:**
   - **Complex Profiles:** Incorporate a balance of flavors—sweet, savory, salty, and acidic—for a sophisticated taste.
   - **Contrasting Elements:** Play with contrasting textures and temperatures for a dynamic culinary experience.

3. **Technique and Presentation:**

   - **Skillful Preparation:** Employ advanced
cooking techniques or methods to showcase
culinary expertise.
   - **Artful Presentation:** Pay attention to plating
and presentation for an aesthetically pleasing dish.

4. **Specialized Dishes:**
   - **Signature Dish:** Include a standout or
signature dish that defines the occasion.
   - **Variety:** Offer a diverse menu with options for
different preferences, including vegetarian or
allergy-friendly choices.

5. **Creative Twists:**
   - **Innovative Combinations:** Experiment with
unique ingredient pairings or unexpected flavor
combinations.
   - **Culinary Creativity:** Showcase inventive
twists on classic dishes for a memorable culinary
experience.

6. **Culinary Themes:**
   - **Cultural Influences:** Infuse elements from
specific cuisines or cultural influences for thematic
cohesion.
   - **Seasonal Themes:** Tailor recipes to suit the
occasion, such as holiday-inspired or celebratory
themes.

7. **Dessert Indulgence:**
   - **Decadent Sweets:** Include a luxurious
dessert that serves as the grand finale.

  - **Gourmet Treats:** Experiment with high-end chocolates, unique pastries, or artisanal sweets.

8. **Wine and Beverage Pairing:**
  - **Thoughtful Pairings:** Consider wine or beverage pairings that complement the meal.
  - **Craft Cocktails:** Introduce handcrafted cocktails that enhance the overall dining experience.

9. **Customization and Personalization:**
  - **Tailored Touches:** Add personalized elements to the dishes or presentation for a bespoke feel.
  - **Customized Portions:** Offer individual or shareable portions to suit the occasion.

10. **Guest Interaction:**
  - **Interactive Elements:** Include dishes with interactive components, such as DIY assembly or tableside preparations.
  - **Engaging Experience:** Aim to create a dining experience that captivates and engages guests.

11. **Attention to Dietary Needs:**
  - **Allergen Considerations:** Accommodate dietary restrictions or allergies to ensure inclusivity.
  - **Health-Conscious Options:** Provide lighter or healthier alternatives for those with specific preferences.

12. **Memorable Elements:**

- **Storytelling Through Food:** Infuse personal or cultural narratives into the culinary experience.
- **Keepsake Elements:** Consider edible keepsakes or mementos for guests to take away.

Recipes for special occasions go beyond mere sustenance; they aim to create lasting memories through exceptional tastes, visual appeal, and a thoughtful approach to the dining experience. Each element, from ingredient selection to presentation, contributes to the overall success of these culinary creations.

HEART-HEALTHY CELEBRATORY DISHES

Certainly! Here are five heart-healthy celebratory dishes with detailed instructions:

1. **Grilled Citrus Salmon with Quinoa Salad:**

Certainly! Here's a delicious recipe for Grilled Citrus Salmon with Quinoa Salad:

Grilled Citrus Salmon:

Ingredients:

- 4 salmon fillets
- Zest of 1 lemon

- Zest of 1 orange
- Juice of 1 lemon
- Juice of 1 orange
- 2 tablespoons olive oil
- 2 cloves garlic, minced
- Salt and pepper to taste

Instructions:

1. **Marinate Salmon:**
   - In a bowl, whisk together lemon zest, orange zest, lemon juice, orange juice, olive oil, minced garlic, salt, and pepper.

Coat Salmon:
   - Place salmon fillets in a dish and pour the citrus marinade over them. Ensure the fillets are well-coated. Allow the flavors to infuse by marinating for a minimum of half an hour.

Grill Salmon:
   - Preheat the grill. Grill the salmon fillets for about 4-5 minutes per side or until cooked to your preferred level of doneness.

Serve:
   - Remove the salmon from the grill and serve it with a side of quinoa salad.

Quinoa Salad:

Ingredients:

- 1 cup quinoa, cooked and cooled
- 1 cup cherry tomatoes, halved
- 1 cucumber, diced
- 1/4 cup red onion, finely chopped
- 1/4 cup feta cheese, crumbled
- 2 tablespoons fresh parsley, chopped
- 3 tablespoons olive oil
- 2 tablespoons balsamic vinegar
- Salt and pepper to taste

Instructions:

1. **Prepare Quinoa:**
   - Cook quinoa according to package instructions. Once cooked, allow it to cool.

Assemble Salad:
   - In a large bowl, combine cooked quinoa, cherry tomatoes, diced cucumber, chopped red onion, crumbled feta cheese, and chopped fresh parsley.

Dress Salad:
   - In a small bowl, whisk together olive oil, balsamic vinegar, salt, and pepper. Pour the dressing over the quinoa salad and toss until well combined.

Serve:
   - Serve the Grilled Citrus Salmon on a bed of Quinoa Salad.

This Grilled Citrus Salmon with Quinoa Salad offers a perfect balance of citrusy flavors, grilled goodness, and a refreshing quinoa salad. It's a nutritious and flavorful dish that's great for a healthy meal.

2. **Stuffed Bell Peppers with Turkey and Black Beans:**

 Certainly! Here's a tasty recipe for Stuffed Bell Peppers with Turkey and Black Beans:

Ingredients:

- 4 large bell peppers, halved and seeds removed
- 1 pound ground turkey
- 1 cup cooked black beans (canned and drained is fine)
- 1 cup cooked quinoa
- 1 cup diced tomatoes
- 1/2 cup corn kernels (fresh or frozen)
- 1/2 cup diced red onion
- 2 cloves garlic, minced
- 1 teaspoon ground cumin
- 1 teaspoon chili powder
- 1/2 teaspoon paprika
- Salt and pepper to taste
- 1 cup of shredded cheese, Monterey Jack, cheddar, or any other type you want
- Fresh cilantro for garnish (optional)

Instructions:

Preheat Oven:
   - Set the oven temperature to 375°F, or 190°C.

Prepare Bell Peppers:
   - Cut the bell peppers in half lengthwise, removing seeds and membranes. Place them in a baking dish.

Cook Turkey:
   - In a skillet over medium heat, cook the ground turkey until browned. Drain any excess fat.

Prepare Filling:
   - In a large bowl, combine the cooked turkey, black beans, cooked quinoa, diced tomatoes, corn, red onion, minced garlic, ground cumin, chili powder, paprika, salt, and pepper. Mix until well combined.

Stuff Bell Peppers:
   - Spoon the filling into each bell pepper half, pressing it down gently. Fill each pepper generously.

Add Cheese:
   - Every filled pepper should have some shredded cheese on top of it.

Bake:

  - Once the oven is preheated, bake the baking
dish covered with foil for 25 to 30 minutes, or until
the peppers are soft.

Garnish:
  - If desired, garnish with fresh cilantro before
serving.

Serve:
  - Serve these delicious Stuffed Bell Peppers with
Turkey and Black Beans as a wholesome and
satisfying meal.

This recipe combines the flavors of lean ground
turkey, black beans, and a variety of spices for a
nutritious and tasty stuffed pepper dish. Enjoy!

3. **Mediterranean Chickpea Salad:**

 Certainly! Here's a refreshing recipe for
Mediterranean Chickpea Salad:

Ingredients:

- Two cans (15 oz each) of rinsed and drained
chickpeas
- 1 cup cherry tomatoes, halved
- 1 cucumber, diced
- 1/2 red onion, finely chopped
- 1/2 cup Kalamata olives, sliced
- 1/2 cup crumbled feta cheese
- 1/4 cup fresh parsley, chopped

- 1/4 cup fresh mint, chopped
- 1/4 cup extra-virgin olive oil
- 2 tablespoons red wine vinegar
- 1 teaspoon dried oregano
- Salt and pepper to taste
- Optional: Lemon wedges for serving

Instructions:

Prepare Chickpeas:
   - Drain and rinse the chickpeas thoroughly. After that, blot them dry using a paper towel.

Assemble Salad:
   - In a large bowl, combine chickpeas, cherry tomatoes, diced cucumber, chopped red onion, sliced Kalamata olives, crumbled feta cheese, chopped parsley, and chopped mint.

Make Dressing:
   - In a small bowl, whisk together extra-virgin olive oil, red wine vinegar, dried oregano, salt, and pepper.

Toss Salad:
   - Pour the dressing over the chickpea mixture and toss gently until all ingredients are well coated.

Chill:
   - To let the flavors combine, cover the bowl and chill it in the refrigerator for at least half an hour.

Serve:
   - Give the salad one more toss before serving,
then taste and adjust the seasoning. Serve with
lemon slices on the side, if desired.

Enjoy:
   - Enjoy this Mediterranean Chickpea Salad as a
light and flavorful dish on its own or as a side dish
to complement your meals.

This salad is bursting with Mediterranean flavors,
featuring chickpeas, fresh vegetables, olives, and
feta cheese. It's perfect for a quick and healthy
lunch or as a side dish for a summer barbecue.

4. **Roasted Vegetable Quiche with Whole Wheat Crust:**

 Certainly! Here's a delicious recipe for Roasted
Vegetable Quiche with Whole Wheat Crust:

Whole Wheat Crust:

Ingredients:

- 1 1/2 cups whole wheat flour
- Half a cup of chilled unsalted butter, sliced into
little cubes
- 1/4 teaspoon salt
- 4-6 tablespoons ice water

Instructions:

Prepare Crust:
   - In a food processor, combine whole wheat flour and salt. Add chilled butter cubes and pulse until the mixture resembles coarse crumbs.

Add Water:
   - One spoonful at a time, gradually add ice water, pulsing after each addition, until the dough starts to come together.

Form Dough:
   - Turn the dough out onto a lightly floured surface and gently knead it a few times until it forms a ball. The ball should be flattened into a disk, covered with plastic wrap, and chilled for a minimum of half an hour.

Roll Out Crust:
   - Adjust the oven's temperature to 190°C, or 375°F. Using a floured surface, roll out the cold dough to fit your pie plate. Transfer the rolled-out crust to the pie dish, pressing it against the edges.

 Pre-bake Crust (Optional):
   - If desired, you can pre-bake the crust for about 10 minutes before adding the filling. This helps prevent a soggy bottom.

Roasted Vegetable Quiche Filling:

Ingredients:

- 1 cup cherry tomatoes, halved
- 1 zucchini, thinly sliced
- 1 red bell pepper, diced
- 1 cup baby spinach
- 6 large eggs
- 1 cup milk (whole or 2%)
- 1 cup grated cheese (you can use Gruyere, cheddar, or your choice).
- Salt and pepper to taste
- 1 tablespoon olive oil

Instructions:

Roast Vegetables:
   - Preheat the oven to 400°F (200°C). Toss cherry tomatoes, zucchini slices, and diced red bell pepper with olive oil. Arrange them evenly on a baking sheet and bake for 15 to 20 minutes, or until they become soft.

Prepare Quiche Filling:
   - In a bowl, whisk together eggs, milk, shredded cheese, salt, and pepper.

Assemble Quiche:
   - Arrange the roasted vegetables and baby spinach over the pre-baked or raw pie crust. Evenly cover the vegetables with the egg mixture.

Bake:

- The quiche should be baked for 35 to 40 minutes in a preheated oven, or until the top is golden brown and the middle is set.

Cool and Serve:
- Allow the quiche to cool for a few minutes before slicing. Serve warm and enjoy!

This Roasted Vegetable Quiche with Whole Wheat Crust is a wholesome and flavorful dish that makes for a delightful brunch or dinner. The combination of roasted veggies, cheesy filling, and a whole wheat crust adds a nutritious twist to a classic quiche.

5. **Herb-Crusted Baked Chicken with Garlic Green Beans:**

Certainly! Here's a tasty recipe for Herb-Crusted Baked Chicken with Garlic Green Beans:

Herb-Crusted Baked Chicken:

Ingredients:

- 4 boneless, skinless chicken breasts
- 2 tablespoons olive oil
- 2 teaspoons dried thyme
- 2 teaspoons dried rosemary
- 1 teaspoon dried oregano
- 1 teaspoon garlic powder
- Salt and pepper to taste
- 1/2 cup breadcrumbs (whole wheat or regular)

Instructions:

Preheat Oven:
   - Set the oven temperature to 400°F, or 200°C.

 Prepare Herb Crust:
   - In a small bowl, mix together dried thyme, dried rosemary, dried oregano, garlic powder, salt, pepper, and breadcrumbs.

Coat Chicken:
   - Brush each chicken breast with olive oil, then coat them evenly with the herb and breadcrumb mixture, pressing the mixture onto the chicken to adhere.

Place on Baking Sheet:
   - Place the herb-crusted chicken breasts on a baking sheet lined with parchment paper.

Bake:
   - Bake in the preheated oven for 20-25 minutes or until the chicken is cooked through and the crust is golden brown.

Garlic Green Beans:

Ingredients:

- 1 pound fresh green beans, trimmed
- 2 tablespoons olive oil

- 3 cloves garlic, minced
- Salt and pepper to taste
- Lemon wedges for serving (optional)

Instructions:

Blanch Green Beans:
   - Bring a pot of water to boil and blanch the green beans for about 2 minutes. Quickly empty and place them in an ice water bath to halt the cooking procedure. Drain again.

Sauté Garlic:
   - In a skillet, heat olive oil over medium heat. Saute the minced garlic for one to two minutes, until it becomes aromatic.

Add Green Beans:
   - Add the blanched green beans to the skillet. Toss them in the garlic-infused oil until well-coated.

Season:
   - To taste, add salt and pepper to the green beans. Cook the beans for a further two to three minutes, or until they are crisp-tender.

Serve:
   - Serve the Herb-Crusted Baked Chicken with Garlic Green Beans. Optionally, squeeze lemon wedges over the green beans for extra freshness.

This Herb-Crusted Baked Chicken with Garlic Green Beans is a flavorful and wholesome meal that's easy to prepare. The combination of aromatic herbs and garlic enhances the chicken, while the green beans add a crisp and vibrant side to the dish. Enjoy!

HOLIDAY FEAST WITH A NUTRITIONAL FOCUS

Creating a holiday feast with a nutritional focus is a wonderful way to celebrate while prioritizing health. Here's a menu with detailed instructions for a wholesome and delicious holiday meal:

1. **Appetizer: Roasted Butternut Squash Soup**

 Certainly! Here's a delicious recipe for Roasted Butternut Squash Soup, perfect as an appetizer:

Ingredients:

- One medium butternut squash that has been chopped, skinned, and seeded
- 1 onion, chopped
- 2 carrots, peeled and chopped
- 2 apples, peeled, cored, and chopped
- 3 cloves garlic, minced
- 2 tablespoons olive oil
- 4 cups vegetable broth

- 1 teaspoon ground cinnamon
- 1/2 teaspoon ground nutmeg
- Salt and pepper to taste
- One cup of optional coconut milk (for creaminess)
- Fresh parsley or chives for garnish

Instructions:

Roast Vegetables:
   - Preheat the oven to 400°F (200°C). Place diced butternut squash, chopped onion, chopped carrots, chopped apples, and minced garlic on a baking sheet. Drizzle with olive oil, toss to coat, and roast in the oven for about 30-35 minutes or until vegetables are tender.

Blend Roasted Vegetables:
   - After roasting, transfer the veggies to a blender. Add vegetable broth, ground cinnamon, ground nutmeg, salt, and pepper. Blend until smooth and creamy.

 Heat Soup:
   - Pour the blended mixture into a pot. Heat the soup over medium heat until it simmers. If you prefer a creamier soup, stir in coconut milk at this stage.

Adjust Seasoning:
   - Taste the soup and adjust the seasoning, adding more salt or pepper if needed.

Serve:
   - Ladle the Roasted Butternut Squash Soup into
bowls. Garnish with fresh parsley or chives.

Enjoy:
   - Serve this warm and comforting soup as an
appetizer, perfect for fall or winter gatherings.

This Roasted Butternut Squash Soup is rich,
flavorful, and has a hint of sweetness from the
roasted vegetables and apples. It's a great way to
start a meal with a comforting and seasonal touch.

2. **Main Course: Herb-Roasted Turkey Breast with Cranberry Chutney**

 Certainly! Here's a delightful recipe for
Herb-Roasted Turkey Breast with Cranberry
Chutney, perfect as a main course:

Herb-Roasted Turkey Breast:

Ingredients:

- 1 bone-in turkey breast (about 4-5 pounds)
- 3 tablespoons olive oil
- 2 teaspoons dried thyme
- 2 teaspoons dried rosemary
- 1 teaspoon dried sage
- Salt and pepper to taste
- 1 cup chicken or turkey broth

Instructions:

Preheat Oven:
   - Set the oven temperature to 375°F, or 190°C.

Prepare Turkey Breast:
   - Using paper towels, pat dry the turkey breast.
Put it inside a roasting pan on a roasting rack.

Herb Rub:
   - In a small bowl, mix together olive oil, dried
thyme, dried rosemary, dried sage, salt, and pepper
to form a herb rub.

Coat Turkey:
   - Rub the herb mixture all over the turkey breast,
ensuring even coverage.

Roast:
   - Fill the roasting pan's bottom with the stock from
the bird or turkey. Roast the turkey breast in the
preheated oven for about 1.5 to 2 hours or until the
internal temperature reaches 165°F (74°C), basting
occasionally with the pan juices.

Rest:
   - Once cooked, let the turkey breast rest for about
15 minutes before slicing.

Cranberry Chutney:

Ingredients:

- 2 cups fresh or frozen cranberries
- 1/2 cup orange juice
- 1/2 cup brown sugar
- 1/4 cup chopped red onion
- 1/4 cup raisins
- 1 teaspoon grated fresh ginger
- 1/4 teaspoon ground cinnamon
- Pinch of salt

Instructions:

Cook Cranberries:
   - In a saucepan, combine cranberries, orange juice, brown sugar, chopped red onion, raisins, grated ginger, ground cinnamon, and a pinch of salt.

Simmer:
   - Bring the mixture to a simmer over medium heat. Cook, stirring occasionally, until the cranberries burst and the chutney thickens (about 15-20 minutes).

Cool:
   - Take the chutney from the stove and let it cool. As it cools, it will get thicker.

Serve:
   - Serve the Herb-Roasted Turkey Breast with a generous spoonful of Cranberry Chutney.

This Herb-Roasted Turkey Breast with Cranberry Chutney is a festive and flavorful main course, perfect for holiday dinners or special occasions. The combination of savory herb-roasted turkey and sweet-tart cranberry chutney creates a delightful harmony of flavors.

3. **Side Dish: Roasted Vegetable Salad with Quinoa**

Absolutely! Here's a tasty recipe for Quinoa and Roasted Vegetable Salad, perfect as a side dish:

Ingredients:

- 1 cup quinoa, rinsed
- 2 cups water or vegetable broth
- 1 medium-sized eggplant, diced
- 1 zucchini, diced
- 1 red bell pepper, diced
- 1 yellow bell pepper, diced
- 1 red onion, sliced
- 3 tablespoons olive oil
- Salt and pepper to taste
- 1/4 cup fresh parsley, chopped
- 1/4 cup feta cheese, crumbled (optional)
- Balsamic vinaigrette dressing (store-bought or homemade)

Instructions:

Preheat Oven:

- Set the oven temperature to 400°F, or 200°C.

Roast Vegetables:
   - In a large bowl, toss diced eggplant, zucchini, red bell pepper, yellow bell pepper, and sliced red onion with olive oil, salt, and pepper. Spread the vegetables evenly on a baking sheet.

Roast:
   - Roast the vegetables in the preheated oven for about 25-30 minutes or until they are tender and slightly caramelized. To ensure consistent cooking, stir the vegetables halfway during the roasting process.

Cook Quinoa:
   - While the vegetables are roasting, rinse the quinoa under cold water. Quinoa should be combined with water or vegetable broth in a saucepan. After bringing to a boil, lower the heat to a simmer, cover, and cook the quinoa for 15 to 20 minutes, or until it is tender and the liquid has been absorbed. Fluff the quinoa with a fork.

Combine:
   - In a large bowl, combine the cooked quinoa and roasted vegetables. Toss gently to mix.

Add Fresh Herbs:
   - Stir in chopped fresh parsley. This adds a burst of freshness to the salad.

Optional: Feta Cheese:
   - If desired, sprinkle crumbled feta cheese over the salad for added creaminess and tanginess.

Dress:
   - Drizzle the quinoa and roasted vegetable salad with balsamic vinaigrette dressing. Toss to coat evenly.

Serve:
   - You can serve the salad warm or at room temperature.

This Quinoa and Roasted Vegetable Salad is a versatile and nutritious side dish that pairs well with various proteins or can be enjoyed on its own. The combination of quinoa, roasted vegetables, and flavorful dressing creates a satisfying and wholesome dish.

4. **Side Dish: Garlic Mashed Cauliflower**

Certainly! Here's a delicious recipe for Garlic Mashed Cauliflower, a healthy and flavorful side dish:

Ingredients:

- 1 large head of cauliflower, cut into florets
- 3 cloves garlic, minced
- 2 tablespoons olive oil
- Salt and pepper to taste

- 1/4 cup grated Parmesan cheese (optional)
- Chopped fresh chives or parsley for garnish

Instructions:

Steam Cauliflower:
  - Place the cauliflower florets in a steamer basket over a pot of simmering water. Steam for about 10-12 minutes or until the cauliflower is tender when pierced with a fork.

Sauté Garlic:
  - While the cauliflower is steaming, heat olive oil in a skillet over medium heat. Add minced garlic and sauté for 1-2 minutes until fragrant. Make sure it doesn't become brown.

Blend Cauliflower:
  - Transfer the steamed cauliflower to a food processor or blender. Add the sautéed garlic and olive oil. Blend until smooth and creamy.

Season:
  - Season the mashed cauliflower with salt and pepper to taste. If you like, you can also stir in grated Parmesan cheese for added flavor.

Garnish:
  - Garnish the garlic mashed cauliflower with chopped fresh chives or parsley.

Serve:

- Serve the Garlic Mashed Cauliflower as a flavorful and low-carb alternative to traditional mashed potatoes.

This Garlic Mashed Cauliflower is a tasty and nutritious side dish that complements a variety of main courses. The garlic adds a savory kick, and the creamy texture makes it a satisfying substitute for mashed potatoes. Enjoy!

5. **Side Dish: Sautéed Green Beans with Almonds**

 Certainly! Here's a simple and flavorful recipe for Sautéed Green Beans with Almonds, a delightful side dish:

Ingredients:

- 1 pound fresh green beans, ends trimmed
- 2 tablespoons olive oil
- 2 cloves garlic, minced
- 1/4 cup sliced almonds
- Salt and pepper to taste
- Lemon wedges for serving (optional)

Instructions:

Blanch Green Beans:
   - Bring a pot of water to boil and add the trimmed green beans. Blanch for about 2 minutes until they are bright green and slightly tender. Put them in an

ice water bath right away to halt the cooking process. Drain and pat dry.

Sauté Garlic and Almonds:
   - Heat the olive oil in a big skillet over medium heat. Add minced garlic and sliced almonds. Sauté for 1-2 minutes until the almonds are lightly toasted and the garlic is fragrant.

Add Green Beans:
   - Add the blanched green beans to the skillet. Toss them in the garlic-infused oil and almonds until well-coated.

 Season:
   - To taste, add salt and pepper to the green beans. Continue to sauté for an additional 2-3 minutes until the beans are tender-crisp.

Serve:
   - Transfer the Sautéed Green Beans with Almonds to a serving dish. Optionally, serve with lemon wedges on the side for a burst of freshness.

Enjoy:
   - Serve this flavorful side dish alongside your favorite main course.

This Sautéed Green Beans with Almonds is a quick and delicious way to elevate green beans. The combination of toasted almonds and garlic adds a nutty richness to the vibrant green beans, creating a tasty and visually appealing side dish.

6. **Dessert: Berry and Greek Yogurt Parfait**

Certainly! Here's a delightful recipe for Berry and Greek Yogurt Parfait, a refreshing and healthy dessert:

Ingredients:

- 1 cup Greek yogurt (plain or vanilla)
- One cup of mixed berries, including raspberries, blueberries, and strawberries
- 2 tablespoons honey or maple syrup
- 1/2 cup granola
- Fresh mint leaves for garnish (optional)

Instructions:

Prepare Greek Yogurt:
  - blend the Greek yogurt and maple syrup in a bowl, stirring to fully blend. Adjust the sweetness to your liking.

Layering:
  - In serving glasses or bowls, start by adding a layer of Greek yogurt at the bottom.

Add Berries:

- Top the yogurt layer with a generous portion of mixed berries.

Repeat Layers:
- Repeat the layering process by adding another layer of Greek yogurt on top of the berries.

Top with Granola:
- Sprinkle a layer of granola over the Greek yogurt. This adds a delightful crunch to the parfait.

Final Layer of Berries:
- Finish off the parfait with a final layer of mixed berries.

Garnish:
- Optionally, garnish the parfait with fresh mint leaves for a burst of color and added freshness.

Serve:
- Serve the Berry and Greek Yogurt Parfait immediately or refrigerate until ready to enjoy.

This Berry and Greek Yogurt Parfait is a delicious and visually appealing dessert that combines the creamy goodness of Greek yogurt with the sweetness of fresh berries and the crunch of granola. It's a healthy and satisfying treat for any occasion.

7. **Beverage: Infused Water with Citrus and Mint**

Certainly! Here's a refreshing recipe for Infused Water with Citrus and Mint, a hydrating and flavorful beverage:

Ingredients:

- 1 lemon, thinly sliced
- 1 lime, thinly sliced
- 1 orange, thinly sliced
- Fresh mint leaves
- Ice cubes
- Water

Instructions:

Prepare Citrus Slices:
   - Wash the lemon, lime, and orange thoroughly. Slice them thinly, keeping the peels on for added flavor.

Assemble Infused Water:
   - In a large pitcher, combine the citrus slices and a handful of fresh mint leaves.

Muddle Mint:
   - Gently muddle the mint leaves with a muddler or the back of a spoon. This helps release the mint's essential oils.

Add Ice Cubes:

- Place ice cubes in the pitcher. This will keep the infused water cool and refreshing.

Fill with Water:
- Pour cold water into the pitcher, covering the citrus slices, mint, and ice.

Stir:
- Give the infused water a gentle stir to mix the flavors.

Refrigerate:
- Let the infused water refrigerate for at least 1-2 hours to allow the flavors to meld.

Serve:
- Serve the Infused Water with Citrus and Mint over ice. Optionally, garnish individual glasses with additional citrus slices and mint leaves.

This Infused Water with Citrus and Mint is a delicious and hydrating beverage, perfect for staying refreshed. The combination of citrus fruits and mint creates a light and revitalizing drink, making it an excellent choice for any time of the day.

This holiday feast is designed with a nutritional focus, incorporating lean protein, whole grains, plenty of vegetables, and healthy fats. It's a balanced and flavorful meal that allows for celebration without compromising on health-conscious choices. Enjoy the feast and the festive spirit!

CONCLUSION

In conclusion, the Heart Disease Cookbook for Women is a comprehensive and empowering resource designed to promote cardiovascular health through mindful nutrition. This cookbook not only addresses the specific dietary needs of women but also emphasizes the importance of a heart-conscious lifestyle.

Starting with an informative introduction, the cookbook delves into the fundamentals of understanding heart health, highlighting the significance of nutrition in preventing heart disease. The exploration of heart-healthy basics provides a solid foundation, guiding women towards making informed choices for their well-being.

The inclusion of essential nutrients for cardiovascular health and detailed explanations on cooking techniques for heart-friendly meals equips women with practical knowledge to enhance their culinary skills while prioritizing heart health. Emphasizing the importance of lifestyle factors, the cookbook seamlessly integrates nutrition into a broader context of overall well-being.

The diverse and delicious recipes, from breakfast boosters to snacks with purpose, offer a range of options that cater to different tastes and preferences. The inclusion of fiber-rich morning starters, low-sodium and nutrient-packed choices, lean proteins, heart-healthy fats, and flavorful vegetable entrées reflects the cookbook's commitment to variety and nutritional balance.

The cookbook further goes beyond recipes by providing lifestyle tips for heart health, reinforcing the idea that a holistic approach involves not only what is on the plate but also daily habits and self-care. The emphasis on physical activity, stress management techniques, and mindful portion control complements the culinary aspect, fostering a well-rounded approach to heart wellness.

In essence, the Heart Disease Cookbook for Women serves as a valuable guide, empowering women to take charge of their cardiovascular health through informed and delicious choices. By combining nutritional insights, practical recipes, and lifestyle guidance, this cookbook strives to be a companion in the journey towards a heart-healthy and fulfilling life for women.

RECAP OF HEART-HEALTHY COOKING PRINCIPLES

In recap, the Heart-Healthy Cookbook for Women is founded on key principles that prioritize cardiovascular well-being through mindful and nutritious cooking. Here's a summary of the heart-healthy cooking principles highlighted in the cookbook:

1. **Understanding Heart Health:**
  - The cookbook begins with an introduction and exploration of essential concepts related to heart health.
  - Emphasis is placed on the significance of a heart-conscious lifestyle, tailored specifically for women's cardiovascular needs.

2. **Importance of Nutrition:**
  - Recognizes the crucial role of nutrition in preventing heart disease.
  - Provides insights into essential nutrients that contribute to cardiovascular health, fostering an understanding of their impact on the body.

3. **Heart-Healthy Basics:**
  - Establishes foundational principles for heart-healthy eating, encompassing whole foods, lean proteins, and nutrient-dense choices.
  - Encourages a balance of essential nutrients, including fiber, vitamins, and minerals.

4. **Cooking Techniques for Heart-Friendly Meals:**
  - Explores cooking methods that enhance flavor and nutrition without compromising heart health.
  - Highlights techniques that reduce the reliance on excessive fats, sodium, and refined sugars.

5. **Essential Nutrients for Cardiovascular Health:**
   - Provides detailed explanations about key nutrients such as omega-3 fatty acids, antioxidants, and fiber.
   - Guides women on incorporating these nutrients into their daily meals for optimal heart health.

6. **Lifestyle Tips for Heart Wellness:**
   - Extends beyond the kitchen to encompass overall well-being.
   - Encourages regular physical activity, stress management techniques, mindful portion control, and other lifestyle factors.

7. **Heart-Healthy Recipes:**
   - Offers a variety of recipes tailored for heart-conscious eating, including breakfast boosters, fiber-rich morning starters, lean proteins, and flavorful vegetable entrées.
   - Promotes diverse and delicious options, ensuring a balanced and satisfying culinary experience.

8. **Snacks with Purpose:**
   - Recognizes the importance of snacks as integral components of a heart-healthy diet.
   - Provides recipes that align with nutritional principles while offering satisfying and purposeful snack options.

9. **Mindful Portion Control:**

- Advocates for mindful eating and portion control to maintain a balanced and healthy diet.
- Empowers women to be conscious of their serving sizes without sacrificing enjoyment.

10. **Holistic Approach to Heart Wellness:**
- Recognizes the interconnectedness of nutrition, physical activity, and stress management in fostering overall heart wellness.
- Encourages women to adopt a holistic and sustainable approach to cardiovascular health.

By adhering to these heart-healthy cooking principles, the cookbook aims to empower women with the knowledge and tools to make informed, flavorful, and heart-conscious choices in their daily culinary endeavors.

EMPOWERING WOMEN TO PRIORITIZE HEART HEALTH

Empowering women to prioritize heart health involves fostering awareness, providing education, and encouraging positive lifestyle changes. Here are key strategies to empower women in prioritizing their cardiovascular well-being:

1. **Educational Resources:**
- Offer accessible and comprehensible educational materials, such as pamphlets, articles,

and online resources, to increase awareness of heart health.
   - Provide information specifically tailored to women, addressing their unique risk factors and symptoms.

2. **Community Workshops and Seminars:**
   - Conduct workshops and seminars focused on heart health, covering topics like nutrition, exercise, stress management, and early detection of heart-related issues.
   - Encourage open discussions to address questions and concerns related to women's heart health.

3. **Personalized Health Assessments:**
   - Encourage women to undergo regular health assessments, including cholesterol checks, blood pressure measurements, and cardiovascular risk assessments.
   - Empower them with personalized insights into their heart health status.

4. **Heart-Healthy Cooking Classes:**
   - Organize cooking classes that emphasize heart-healthy recipes and cooking techniques.
   - Provide practical demonstrations on preparing nutritious and delicious meals tailored to women's cardiovascular needs.

5. **Support Networks:**

- Establish support networks where women can share experiences, challenges, and successes related to heart health.
- Create a sense of community to foster encouragement and motivation.

6. **Physical Activity Initiatives:**
- Promote physical activity through inclusive initiatives like group fitness classes, walking groups, or dance sessions.
- Highlight the benefits of regular exercise for heart health and overall well-being.

7. **Stress Management Workshops:**
- Conduct stress management workshops that teach effective coping strategies, such as mindfulness, meditation, and relaxation techniques.
- Empower women to manage stress as a crucial aspect of heart health.

8. **Holistic Lifestyle Approach:**
- Advocate for a holistic approach to health that considers nutrition, physical activity, mental health, and sleep patterns.
- Encourage women to adopt balanced and sustainable lifestyle practices.

9. **Regular Health Checkups:**
- Promote the importance of regular health checkups, screenings, and preventive measures.
- Reinforce the significance of early detection and intervention in maintaining heart health.

10. **Online Health Platforms:**
   - Leverage online platforms to disseminate information, resources, and tools related to heart health.
   - Provide interactive features, such as forums, webinars, and virtual support groups, to connect women with healthcare professionals and peers.

11. **Cultural Sensitivity:**
   - Tailor empowerment initiatives to be culturally sensitive, recognizing diverse perspectives and traditions related to women's health.
   - Address cultural factors that may impact lifestyle choices and healthcare seeking behavior.

12. **Celebration of Heart-Healthy Achievements:**
   - Acknowledge and celebrate women who make positive changes in their lifestyle for heart health.
   - Share success stories to inspire others within the community.

By implementing these strategies, we can empower women to take charge of their heart health, fostering a proactive and informed approach to well-being. Through education, community support, and accessible resources, women can prioritize heart health and cultivate a lifestyle that contributes to long-term cardiovascular wellness.